DO THIS ☑

& LIVE

HEALTHY

10

SIMPLE KEYS THAT CURE

DO THIS ☑ & LIVE HEALTHY

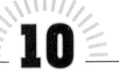

10
SIMPLE KEYS THAT CURE

DON VERHULST, MD

SILOAM

Most CHARISMA HOUSE BOOK GROUP products are available at special quantity discounts for bulk purchase for sales promotions, premiums, fund-raising, and educational needs. For details, write Charisma House Book Group, 600 Rinehart Road, Lake Mary, Florida 32746, or telephone (407) 333-0600.

Do THIS AND LIVE HEALTHY by Don VerHulst, MD
Published by Siloam
Charisma Media/Charisma House Book Group
600 Rinehart Road
Lake Mary, Florida 32746
www.charismahouse.com

Cover design by Justin Evans
Design Director: Bill Johnson

Visit the author's website at www.DrDonMD.com.

AUTHOR NOTE: Dr. Don VerHulst completed his doctor of medicine degree at Wayne State University. Feeling called by the Lord to be a health educator rather than a practicing physician, Dr. Don chose not to become licensed to practice medicine.

Library of Congress Cataloging-in-Publication Data:
An application to register this book for cataloging has been submitted to the Library of Congress.
International Standard Book Number: 978-1-61638-826-3
E-book ISBN: 978-1-61638-827-0

Portions of this book were published as *Ten Keys That Cure* by Don VerHulst, MD, ISBN 978-0-98209-080-0, copyright © 2008.

12 13 14 15 16— 987654321
Printed in the United States of America

DEDICATION

To the one, true, living God
in whom we live and move and have our being!
— Acts 17:28; Jeremiah 9:23–24

CONTENTS

SECTION II: DR. DON'S EASY REFERENCE GUIDE FOR COMMON HEALTH PROBLEMS

FOREWORD

I HAVE KNOWN DR. Don VerHulst for well over twenty years. At one time an atheist, after making the decision to follow Christ he caught fire for God. He and Susie have been members of our church for many years; we have ministered in the States and overseas together.

Dr. Don's approach to biblical health is sound and is very easy to incorporate into your life and family. His book *Do This and Live Healthy* is filled with biblical principles that have been a blessing to me, my wife, Jeanie, and our family. I know they will bless you and your family as well.

—DUANE VANDER KLOK
SENIOR PASTOR, RESURRECTION LIFE CHURCH,
GRANDVILLE, MICHIGAN
FOUNDER, RESURRECTION LIFE CHURCH INTERNATIONAL

GOD WANTS YOU TO ENROLL IN HIS PERFECT HEALTH PLAN

Ever hear the story about the scientist who was determined to scale the Mountain of Truth? He acquired all the knowledge humanly possible and struggled mightily through untold hardships to reach the summit, only to find a theologian already sitting on the peak when he arrived. Though he had nearly killed himself with exertion, the theologian looked as if he were enjoying a day at the beach.

I lived that story. I was that scientist. Early in life I decided that through knowledge and yeoman-like effort I could instill meaning in my life and transform others' lives for the better. Applying myself to medical school, I spent years in intensive study, sacrificing my time and sanity to meet the rigors of a grueling schedule. In 1982 I earned my medical degree. Little did I know that an MD wouldn't bring me the happiness and fulfillment that I had been seeking.

TAKE CARE OF YOUR "EARTH SUIT"

God created us as three-part beings: spirit, soul, and body. All three parts were a mess by the time I finished med school. An atheist without any hope, I had stuffed my mind full of medical jargon and tradition. I lived on caffeine, junk food, and adrenaline. Though I never exercised, I looked like a pencil and couldn't gain weight. Running day and night, I was a living contradiction—a doctor who didn't take care of his health. Despite my sorry physical and spiritual state, I was convinced that I was well on my way to reaching the pinnacle of life. Then one night my car battery died, and the scientist met the theologian.

"What do you believe in?"

Cough. Sputter. Cough. At 4:00 a.m. in the freezing cold that had settled over the Detroit Metropolitan Airport, starting my car looked hopeless. That is, until a gentleman approached in his truck, stopped, and offered a jump start. After retrieving his jumper cables, he offered to let me sit in his warm vehicle while he charged my battery. Once the cables were hooked up, he climbed in too. Out of the blue he asked me a question I wasn't expecting: "What do you believe in?"

Though that struck me as an odd question to ask in a frozen parking lot in the predawn hours, I thought, "Well, this guy's jumping my car battery, so if he wants to talk about the cost of tea in China, all right then, let's talk!" So I replied, "Well, I've heard about God and Jesus, but I don't believe all that. I'm an atheist."

In the past that statement either riled people up or scared them into silence. This late-night theologian acted just like I believe Jesus would have. After listening quietly to everything I had to say after that blunt, introductory declaration, he nodded his head and asked a simple question: "Have you ever sinned?"

"Oh yeah! I'm the grand champion sinner!" I said quickly, smiling. (Isn't it interesting that I was an atheist and I still knew I had sinned?

The scientific Bible

The more I studied the Bible, the more particular verses would jump out at me, particularly ones containing divine principles about the physical body, health, and healing. In all my years of medical studies the Bible was certainly the last book I would have considered a leading textbook on physiology. However, I discovered that God's Word is absolutely the most current, most accurate text on every subject, including physiology and all the sciences. The more scientists and medical experts discover about our "earth suits"—these flesh-and-blood bodies we live in while we're on this planet—the more amazed they are at how the Bible's physiological statements keep proving true. Every divine principle Scripture has stated about physical health and healing is steadfastly accurate.

It is the exact opposite in the academic arena where I come from. Medical advice changes constantly, from year to year—sometimes from month to month. The simplest questions, such as whether a person should take an aspirin daily for heart health, provoke hot debates that appear to never get settled.

Given this reality, I felt delighted to learn that God's Word provides a rock-solid foundation that doesn't shift with the winds of time. It covers every area of life. As a physician I was particularly interested to discover that it provides a pattern for good health. I am continually amazed at the simplicity and practicality of God's health plan. The Bible contains a blueprint that we can easily follow to build health and healing in our physical bodies.

I still have that desire to make my life count for something and to benefit others with what I have learned. That is why I travel, teach, and write about God's perfect health plan for us. I want everyone to enjoy His physical blessings! Good health is vitally important if we hope to enjoy the abundant life God promises and to accomplish

Looking back, I can see now that God had been working in heart.)

"Would you like to be forgiven for your sins?" he asked.

"You mean every wrong thing I've ever done would just be gon replied, somewhat amazed by his question.

"That's right," this stranger affirmed. "Would you like that?"

"That's not even remotely possible," I thought. "We're play hypothetical game here, but at least my car battery's charging.

After debating with myself for a few moments, I responded, would have to be a fool not to want that! Who wouldn't want

"Then ask Jesus to come into your heart and be Lord of yor he said.

Now, as an atheist, I had no idea how to pray, but sud realized this guy knew the truth I had struggled for years tc Though I only said one word—yes—I meant it with every my being. Without warning it felt like the world had shifte my feet.

Immediately the God whom I hadn't even believed ir second before spoke to me as clearly as I've ever heard anyo life. Chills ran up and down my spine, as if He had stepped truck and were staring me in the eye. "Every word of th true," He said. "Even the hairs of your head are all numbe

Those words reminded me of a Bible verse I had heard boy: "The very hairs of your head are all numbered" (Matt was such a revelation that the God of the universe knev me (as He does about each of us). I realized that if He kn well, He must have a specific plan for me. For the next all I wanted to do was study God's Word and learn more He had designed for me to do.

His purposes. No matter what frustrations you have faced with poor health, obesity, or hereditary diseases, I assure you that you can enjoy the good health Scripture talks about.

In Hebrew, *health* means "medicine." God's Word is medicine to your body, soul, and spirit. His divine principles will help you live—really live—and burst with vitality. Trust me as a physician, the medicine we are about to take from His Word is the very best that's available to promote your physical health. Best of all, it is not hard to take!

Good health in God's Word

When I refer to abundant life in regards to your health, I mean more than just the absence of disease. Good health means being full of energy and enthusiasm for living. Christians who take care of their earth suits wake up in the morning full of life spiritually and physically. They have a spring in their step. They overflow with the energy needed to go out and do God's will. They aren't weighed down by a negative outlook, excess weight, or fearful apprehension about what the day will bring.

The more I studied Scripture from a physician's perspective, the more I saw a blueprint emerge that we can follow to achieve and enjoy good health. God's blueprint is marvelous in its simplicity yet profound in its design. Simple yet profound may sound a bit cliché, but it sums up the perfect health plan God provides us in His Word.

Many people give up on the hope of ever experiencing good health because they think that they will face too many rules to follow, too many activities to add to their overburdened schedules, and too many details to assimilate into a biblical nutrition plan. Although they feel guilty about their bleak physical condition, too many decide that pursuing good health is just too complicated because they feel overwhelmed.

I hope to reach millions with the message that God's simple yet profound health plan *will work* for them. Rather than wrestling with complicated programs or agonizing over all the things they shouldn't do or shouldn't eat, people can get healthy and stay healthy by "doing the dos." Rather than focusing on negatives, those who "do the dos"—follow the simple principles the Bible recommends for good health—will reap a huge harvest of physical benefits.

Why "do the dos"?

Your body is *by far* your most valuable worldly possession. You can own five homes, a cottage, a castle, and a yacht, but if you don't have a healthy body, you can't enjoy any of them! And if you stagger with weight or are in pain as you walk down the street, you can't serve the Lord too well on earth either. This is why taking care of your body is such an important part of serving Him.

The apostle Paul urged in Romans 12:1, "I beseech you therefore, brethren, by the mercies of God, that you present your bodies a living sacrifice, holy, acceptable to God, which is your reasonable service." He also taught in 1 Corinthians 6:13 that our bodies are for the Lord and the Lord is for our bodies. The New Living Translation ends that verse with the phrase, "The Lord cares about our bodies." I am glad that He cares! It is good to have Him on our side when it comes to good health.

The Gospels of Matthew, Mark, Luke, and John often relate that Jesus healed *all* the sick that were brought to Him. And whenever a sick person professed a belief that Jesus could heal *if* He were willing, Jesus always replied, "I am!" It pleases me to know that "Jesus Christ is the same yesterday, today, and forever" (Heb. 13:8) and that He still wants His children healed, whole, and feeling great.

Why else should we "do the dos"? They keep us out of trouble! As

Psalm 94:12–13 puts it: "Blessed is the man whom You instruct, O Lord, and teach out of Your law, that You may give him rest from the days of adversity." When we apply the principles about our health contained in Scripture, we are better equipped to avoid the adversity of serious illness and pain.

"The way of transgressors is hard," warns Proverbs 13:15 (kjv). Those who transgress scriptural health principles and neglect their earth suits will be the first to tell you this is true. Anyone with a debilitating illness brought on by self-neglect or anyone undergoing a serious operation to correct a problem they could have prevented with healthier living habits will assure you that the trouble they live with wasn't worth it. If they could only do it over again, they certainly would!

The health equation

My very first day in medical school I sat in a classroom of eager young medical students facing our first instructor in our first lecture. "Before I was a physician, I was an engineer," he began, "and when I was an engineer and a machine broke down, I had to go out and fix it. Then we tried the machine. If it worked, I got the credit."

Looks of confusion came over our faces. We were a bit unsure of what that statement had to do with medicine. Thankfully he went on to explain: "Then I became a physician. As a physician, when the human body 'machine' breaks down, I watch the machine fix itself—and I still get the credit!"

I give that professor high marks for credibility. I have never seen a truer statement in action. Since earning my doctor of medicine degree, I have seen this play out repeatedly. Our bodies are indeed marvelously and wonderfully made (Ps. 139:14). Our bodies *do* fix themselves. They are naturally designed to function efficiently and fight off disease. And when necessary, repair themselves.

We are already built to enjoy great health—but we too have a part to play. Thomas Edison, whose inventions included the electric light bulb, the phonograph, and the first motion picture camera, recognized this when he observed, "The doctor of the future will give no medicine, but will interest her or his patients in the care of the human frame, in a proper diet, and in the cause and prevention of disease."[1]

When we do our part to care for our human frames the biblical way, we give our bodies what they need to function well and to fight off and prevent disease. This is precisely what I teach people to do. The first principle I teach is what I call the health equation, which goes like this:

Detoxification + balancing the immune system = great health

If we will pay attention to detoxification of our bodies while balancing the immune system, we will become far healthier and stay that way. Detoxification, or detox for short, simply means keeping junk out of our bodies and cleansing it of any junk already inside. It is important to "cleanse ourselves from everything that contaminates and defiles body and spirit" (2 Cor. 7:1, AMP). In doing so, we are best equipped to serve God and carry out His plans for us. In the chapters that follow, I will suggest positive steps to take to detox—I think of it as "dejunking"—our bodies by focusing on nutritional, natural foods.

Balancing our immune system is also crucial because the immune system fights off and prevents disease. An immune system strengthened and built up by good health habits can handle any kind of attack that comes at it, whether from an outside source such as a virus or an inside source, such as cancer cells.

Waging war on disease

The tools I recommend are ten keys the Lord showed me about health as I began to study Scripture from a physician's perspective. I call them "Dr. Don's Ten Keys That Cure." Because I have gleaned these keys from the pages of God's Word, they can provide benefits to everyone, whether you are in good health or fighting fatigue, obesity, or sickness.

If you already enjoy good health, they will safeguard it and ensure that you continue to enjoy it. If you are dealing with disease, they will help you detoxify your body and stabilize your immune system so you can begin to balance the health equation in your favor.

In the next ten chapters I will identify these ten keys and examine each one in depth. You will discover how easy they are to learn and apply. As part of my exploration I will discuss specific "dos" in order to put them into practice. These ten keys are modeled throughout both the Old Testament and New Testament. I will show you Jesus Himself followed them in His daily routines. My hope and prayer for you is that as you follow them, you will reap the blessing of great health that God's Word said you were meant to enjoy as long as you are on this earth.

TEN KEYS
THAT CURE

CHAPTER 1

KEY 1:
LEARN TO RELAX LIKE THE LORD

L EARN TO RELAX" is the first and one of the most important of my Ten Keys That Cure. Stress is arguably the number one enemy of the immune system. By stress I don't mean money troubles, issues with your boss, or arguments with your spouse. Those are stressors. Stress is your body's reaction to these stressors.

To briefly explain, God instilled in you a sympathetic nervous system and a parasympathetic nervous system; the latter is the resting system that slows your heart rate and helps you relax. The sympathetic nervous system governs "fight-or-flight" reactions to stressors, meaning it can stress your body. How? By increasing your heart rate, blood pressure, respiration, nutritional needs, and hormonal activity, all in response to some stimuli or stressor. The body goes on "red alert" when this system kicks in. It is good to have a bodily system set up to help you survive—we all need that in certain situations. However, you were never designed to run continually in a state of emergency.

Things happen during a sympathetic nervous system reaction that are not healthy over the long haul. Thinking it needs to focus on *survival*, your body temporarily neglects other important functions.

At least the reaction is designed to be temporary. Under stress your body doesn't think it has time to digest your food properly; when it shifts to other tasks, you don't get all the nutrition you need. Because your body focuses on survival, it neglects your immune system and doesn't fight cancer, infections, and traumas. Gearing up, your body releases fight-or-flight hormones such as adrenaline to aid you in this struggle.

Trouble is, God didn't design humans to continually function under those kinds of extreme reactions. Have you ever heard the saying: "You can't live on adrenaline?" That is true. A continual adrenaline rush will put your health into a long downhill slide. Even so millions of people run around in highly stressed states day after day. Our modern lifestyles set us up to live that way. Before long we think it's normal. That is, until it negatively affects our health.

My wife, Susan, had to learn how to relax the hard way. For a long time she worked outside the home as a popular DJ at a local radio station while also raising our children. To say she woke up on the run doesn't fully yield the picture of her hectic days.

"After I made sure the kids were cared for, I ran out the door, ran to work to record a program, and then ran to the studio in the mall," she recalls. "I ran to the car wash after work and the grocery store after that. Then I ran and got the kids. At home they would start asking, 'What are we going to do?' or saying, 'Let's do this…let's do that,' and quickly we would be off and running again. It's easy to get overstressed and forget about the Sabbath rest—or resting in God at all."

Even now she fights this tendency to race around. Often I can slow her down with a simple question: Have you prayed about whatever is on your mind—all those things on your plate? "That stops me cold," she admits. "We forget to come to God with our burdens and our busyness because we're trying to do it all—and it's making many of us sick!"

One reason I married Susan was because of her high-energy enthusiasm for life. Back in college part of her drive came from caffeine-laden colas and sugar-laden snacks. So when it came to getting balanced nutrition, she was no better than me. Today we live much differently, striving to eat God-made foods that will produce needed energy. In addition to eating right, we also attempt to relax. For some of us that's harder than for others. Yet *learning to relax* is the first of my Ten Keys That Cure.

FOUR-SIX IT!

How do you relax? I advise people to "four-six it." Philippians 4:6 outlines the biblical approach to stress-relief: "Be anxious for nothing, but in everything by prayer and supplication, with thanksgiving, let your requests be made known to God." I love how God not only tells us what not to do, but He also tells us what to do! He says to make *your* requests known to Him. You get to choose your requests. So go ahead and tell Him what you need.

That is a novel idea for many. You would be surprised how many people look at me like a calf at a new gate when I ask them, "Have you made your requests known to God?" It's a wonderful stress buster. Try it! It will settle you down. I like the way The Message version of Philippians 4:6–7 puts it:

> Don't fret or worry. Instead of worrying, pray. Let petitions and praises shape your worries into prayers, letting God know your concerns. Before you know it, a sense of God's wholeness, everything coming together for good, will come and settle you down. It's wonderful what happens when Christ displaces worry at the center of your life.

Continual anxiety or worry is hard on your physiological system—and the rest of you! The crazy thing about worry is that most scenarios we worry about never even come to pass. Famous nineteenth-century author and humorist Mark Twain reportedly once said, "I have been through some terrible things in my life, some of which actually happened."[1]

Sound familiar? We can concentrate on so many what-ifs that it leaves us much less time and energy to deal with life's gritty realities. By worrying, we put ourselves through mental and emotional strains without realizing that they might never even happen. This is why Jesus counseled people: "Therefore do not worry about tomorrow, for tomorrow will worry about its own things. Sufficient for the day is its own trouble" (Matt. 6:34). It may help to recognize that, physiologically, our bodies don't know if the stressors we dwell on are actually happening or not. Either way the body's negative reaction to stress is the same. This is why worrying can literally make us sick.

Let's take a minute to do a little stress-relief. Try some "four-sixing it" right now; it is a great immune-system-stimulating, health-giving activity. Prop this book open with something and put your hands out in front of you, palms up. Visualize all your worries, all the "stuff" in your life—all you are praying about and all you forgot to pray about—in a pile in your hands. Toss everything on the pile (some of us will have bigger piles). On the count of three lift both hands toward heaven while "casting all your care upon Him, for He cares for you" (1 Pet. 5:7). One, two, three...offer your cares to God. Don't put your hands down until you're sure they're empty! Believe in His perfect will in all your circumstances. Don't bring that pile of cares back to earth again. Leave it at His feet where it belongs.

I promise you, your immune system is working better right now than it was a minute ago. You probably feel better too. You can four-six it any time and as often as you want! People may think you've lost your mind when they see you throwing your hands up to heaven, but that's OK. You have the mind of Christ. Whenever you four-six it, you're following the biblical approach to stress relief and strengthening your immune system.

JOY EQUALS STRENGTH

Another relaxation technique is so simple many people miss it, yet it is foundational to enjoying lasting peace. Be joyful. That's it. Rejoice in life. "Don't be dejected and sad, for the joy of the LORD is your strength!" (Neh. 8:10, NLT). The Bible equates joy with strength. If you want a strong immune system and health in other areas, let the Lord fill you with His joy.

Refuse to allow joy killers into your life. Your own words are vital in this. As Proverbs 15:23 says, "A man has joy by the answer of his mouth." Or you have the opposite—your words can bring you sorrow. Align your words with God's Word and speak *positively*. Some people think they are praying when they are really complaining. Realize that God already knows every problem you face. He already has an answer and a plan. So instead of telling God about your problems, tell your problems about God.

Jesus told us to *speak to* the mountains in our lives, not *talk about* them. Tell your mountain to be removed in Jesus's name (Matt. 17:20). If you knew what wonders God has waiting for you on the other side, you would move your mountain in a hurry. Besides, mountains know other mountains. So if you don't tell your mountain to be removed, pretty soon you will have a mountain range, one built with your own complaints or negative words. It's much better to use the positive approach and be joyful.

Cast your cares to heaven and cultivate a joyful heart. In other words, chill out and cheer up! Learning to relax is the first and foremost key to good health. God holds you in the palm of His hand, and He is always on your side. It's the devil who comes to steal, kill, and destroy. Jesus came so that you could enjoy abundant life to the fullest! (See John 10:10.)

LAUGH UNTO THE LORD

Remember there is joy in laughter, so laugh a lot. As Proverbs 17:22 advises, "A merry heart does good, like medicine." Doctors always like that verse since it implies that medicine does good; sometimes medicine can do good, so long as it's taken with your Gos-pills (the gospel message of the good news). Look at The Amplified translation: "A happy heart is good medicine and a cheerful mind works healing, but a broken spirit dries up the bones." Don't walk around crushed and broken when there's healing in Jesus Christ for your every wound. Cheer up at that thought, for a cheerful mind works healing! "Rejoice in the Lord always: and again I say, Rejoice" (Phil. 4:4, KJV).

In our church's healing class we sometimes do "laughter therapy" because laughter breaks down a major stress hormone. Stress hormones bathe our brains in acid. Most of us experience enough issues without having acidic brains that deteriorate quickly and open the door to all kinds of diseases. So we practice laughing our way into joy. Sometimes we have to start with a "laugh of faith," but that's all right—it works. Try it. Do five seconds of laughter therapy now. It will probably turn into at least thirty seconds or more. Once you start, joy just bubbles up inside. You will feel better afterward.

Around our busy household it's gotten so that I recognize my wife's laugh of faith now. I'll hear Susan's "ha-ha-ha" coming from some other part of the house. That makes me laugh because I know she is trying to make the best of something that is probably not very funny. When I do, I get into agreement with her. So do the kids! One time grape juice went flying all over the kitchen table, the curtains, and the floor. I heard Susan's halfhearted "ha-ha-ha" coming from that direction. The kids probably were thinking, "We're in for it now!" After a shocked second, I heard them all join in. No doubt they thought keeping Mom laughing was a better alternative than giving her time to survey the disaster area.

Laughter breaks your focus away from your problems and literally strengthens every system, cell, and organ in your body. My kids know it covers a multitude of sins—even splattering grape juice all over the kitchen. It is amazing that the average adult laughs only fifteen times a day, while the average child laughs between two hundred and four hundred times. My kids laugh constantly. They are full of joy! That keeps their stress hormones from acidifying their brains.

A joyful spirit is healthy and healing: researchers have shown that laughter does the following:

- Relaxes the whole body by relieving physical tension and stress, which relaxes your muscles for up to forty-five minutes.

- Boosts the immune system by decreasing stress hormones and increasing immune cells and infection-fighting antibodies.

- Triggers the release of endorphins, which are your body's "feel good" chemicals; this can temporarily relieve pain.

- Protects the heart by improving blood flow and the functioning of blood vessels, protecting against heart attack and other cardiovascular disease.[2]

In 2005 doctors from the University of Maryland Medical Center released a study that verified the positive impact of laughter on heart health. It involved volunteers who watched both a laughter-provoking movie and a film that produced mental stress. With the amusing films, laughter appeared to cause the tissue that forms the inner lining of blood vessels—the endothelium—to expand in order to increase blood flow. But when volunteers watched one that produced mental stress, their blood vessel lining developed an unhealthy response that reduced blood flow. That confirmed previous studies that suggested a link between mental stress and narrowing of blood vessels.

"The endothelium is the first line in the development of atherosclerosis or hardening of the arteries, so, given the results of our study, it is conceivable that laughing may be important to maintain a healthy endothelium, and reduce the risk of cardiovascular disease," said principal investigator Michael Miller, MD, the center's director of preventive cardiology. "At the very least, laughter offsets the impact of mental stress, which is harmful to the endothelium."[3]

Listen, if experts outside the church are seeing the value of people laughing themselves healthy, it is time to hop on that bandwagon!

CHAPTER 2

KEY 2:
GET TO BED ON TIME:
SLEEP AND THE GREAT HEALER

IN MY CLASSES and seminars, as soon as I mention my second key to good health, "Get to bed on time," chuckles and twitters inevitably echo across the room. It makes me wonder if people think they are reverting to the laughter therapy I talk about in key number one and are using laughter to combat the stress they feel about not getting enough sleep.

Driving while sleepy can be deadly. Don't just take my word for it though. A recent study conducted by the AAA Foundation for Traffic Safety estimated that 17 percent of fatal crashes—or 4,400 a year—are caused by sleepy drivers. The study analyzed crash data from the National Highway Traffic Safety Administration for a ten-year period starting in 1999. Says AAA foundation president Peter Kissinger, "It slows your reaction time and it impairs your judgment."[1]

Driving while sleepy is no laughing matter: "driving under the influence" of sleep deprivation can be as dangerous as driving under the influence of alcohol. In fact, after twenty-four hours of sleeplessness, you are just as impaired behind the wheel of a car as if you were legally drunk. It doesn't even take twenty-four hours for sleep deprivation to begin affecting your driving ability. That can start to happen after seventeen sleepless hours.

Although they don't make the kind of headlines that drunk-driving fatalities do, sleep-deprived accidents are just as deadly. Recently an Illinois attorney secured a $1.2 million judgment from a trucking company after computer data showed one of its driver who plowed into a station wagon, killing five people, had maintained his forty-seven-mile-per-hour speed for six seconds after the accident—a sign he had fallen asleep.[2]

Such mishaps made headlines across the nation in 2011. In Virginia the crash of a tour bus that claimed four lives turned into a criminal investigation after the driver was charged with reckless driving, with investigators basing their theory that fatigue was behind the early-morning fatalities.[3] In California a twenty-three-year-old sleepy driver reportedly drifted into a concrete rail in the center divider, striking an SUV and causing serious injuries to an elderly couple in the vehicle.[4] The coroner in Anderson County, South Carolina, said the driver of a semitrailer fell asleep at the wheel and caused the crash that claimed his life and two others.[5]

Concerns about sleepy drivers have been around for years. In 2003 New Jersey passed the first state law criminalizing drowsy driving. "Maggie's Law" was named for a college student who died after a man who had gone thirty hours without sleep swerved across three lanes of traffic and struck her vehicle head on.[6]

The National Sleep Foundation took a poll in 2009 that showed as many as 1 percent, or 1.9 million drivers, had a car crash or near miss during the previous year. An astonishing 54 percent (105 million) of drivers admitted driving while drowsy at least once. Says Thomas Balkin, chairman of the foundation, "People underestimate how tired they are and think that they can stay awake by sheer force of will. This is a risky misconception. Would there be 1.9 million fatigue-related crashes or near misses if people were good at assessing their own ability to drive when fatigued?"[7]

Given this reality, make sure you are well rested as much as possible, especially if you are going on a long trip. Whenever you climb into a car, thank God—out loud—for safe travel. I especially like to speak this paraphrase of Psalm 91:10–11: "No evil shall happen to me, for God has given His angels charge over me."

GETTING ADEQUATE SLEEP

Getting adequate sleep involves a lot more than avoiding fatal accidents on the highway. It is a key to good health that will pay dividends well into your senior years. Rest time is restoration time. These days most of us have no idea what it is like to wake up feeling restored after a proper night of rest. Yet I cannot overemphasize the simple—and profound—benefits of a good night's sleep.

How beneficial is it to get to bed on time? Actuarial figures from insurance companies show that people who function for more than seven days on five hours of sleep a night (or less) increase their risk of death from all causes by 700 percent! In addition, studies have shown that people who average less than six hours a night don't live as long as people who sleep seven or more hours. As I said in the introduction, people who take care of their earth suit wake up full of life, spiritually and physically. While neglecting your body may not keep you out of heaven, it may well send you there faster. Not getting sufficient rest can literally kill you.

Our bodies require between six and eight hours of good rest every night. Consistency and timing make a world of difference in how you feel and how you function when you wake up. Studies show that the hours from 10:00 p.m. until 2:00 a.m. are the most healing, restorative hours to rest. Don't miss them. From 10:00 p.m. until midnight your sleep is *four times* more restorative than the hours you sleep after midnight.

This restorative rest includes your stomach, which needs good rest every night too. If you get plenty of sleep but still wake up tired, maybe you aren't letting your stomach rest at night. Have you ever noticed that eating a big meal right before bedtime can disturb your sleep or even keep you awake? A simple solution: Don't load up your stomach before bed so that it has to keep working hard all night to digest nocturnal snacks. Instead, follow the maxim "Eat like a king at breakfast, a prince at lunch, and a pauper at dinner." It will do your stomach and sleep habits a world of good.

In 1735 Ben Franklin cited another maxim in his famous *Poor Richard's Almanac*: "Early to bed and early to rise, makes a man healthy, wealthy, and wise."[8] That still makes good sense. God made it easy for us to figure out when to sleep and when to rise. He gave the bright light of sun for the daytime and the lesser lights of the moon and stars for the night. When God's bright light goes down for the night, you go down. When it rises, you rise.

Ben Franklin was right—it is healthy and wise to sleep when God meant us to sleep. Psalm 127:2 says God "gives His beloved sleep." The Amplified version says, "He gives [blessings] to His beloved in their sleep." Beloved child of God, He can't give you sleep and bless you if you won't go to bed on time!

GOD TOOK TIME FOR R AND R

After creating Planet Earth, God Himself took time for rest and relaxation (R and R). The first book of the Bible, Genesis, tells us so. God finished His creative works on earth in six days, checked them over, and saw that they were good. "And on the seventh day God ended His work which He had done; and He rested on the seventh day from all His work which He had done. And God blessed (spoke good of) the seventh day, set it apart as His own, and hallowed it, because on it God rested from all His work which He had created and done" (Gen. 2:2-3, AMP). Some people feel guilty if they take time for R and R, whether that means getting enough sleep at night or allowing for a day of rest on the weekends. Stress, financial worries, or the hectic pace of modern life so overwhelms them that they cannot slow down enough to restore their bodies, minds, and spirits. God "spoke good of" that seventh day of rest though. Later in the Ten Commandments He instructed Moses and the Israelites to rest from all their labors on the seventh day.

God felt so strongly about R and R that He declared the Sabbath holy and decreed, "Whoever does any work on the Sabbath day, he shall surely be put to death" (Exod. 31:15). If that law were in effect today, most of us would likely be struck dead. However, our focus shouldn't be on trying to keep a legalistic set of rules about never working on Sunday (besides, Seventh Day Adventists would immediately disagree with your choice of days). This commandment illustrates the crucial nature of R and R. If God Himself took time off and made this a law for His chosen people, the Israelites, don't you think we ought to make it a priority as well? When properly rested, we will be more productive in body, mind, and spirit.

Jesus knew the importance of R and R. He had a whole world to save, yet look what He did: "Now in the morning, having risen a long while before daylight, He went out and departed to a solitary place; and there He prayed" (Mark 1:35). This one verse contains a whole health seminar and is worth a closer look. Remember the saying that caught fire in the 1990s in the evangelical world: "What would Jesus do?" (WWJD). Here is a saying I like even better: "Do what Jesus did." In other words, "do the dos" as Jesus did in Mark 1:35, and you will go a long way toward experiencing biblical health.

Jesus got to bed on time.

How do I know? Typically, people don't get up early unless they get to bed on time; Jesus consistently got up early. He also consistently went to a solitary place—a peaceful place where He could be alone with God—and prayed. Making time for yourself is vital in learning to relax. You need some time alone and some time with just you and God. That is the best kind of R and R!

He got exercise and prayed.

Notice a couple other things about Jesus's morning routine. Mark says He rose up and went out—in other words, He exercised His physical body. He could have talked to His heavenly Father while lying on His mat (or wherever He slept; the Scriptures tell us sometimes He had nowhere to lay His head). Instead, He got out of bed and took a walk. He walked until He found a peaceful place.

He breathed fresh air and enjoyed the sunshine.

I think He must have watched many glorious sunrises while He prayed. By getting exercise, breathing fresh air, and enjoying sunshine, Jesus practiced three health keys that I will look at in greater detail in coming chapters. Jesus was in the habit of ministering to His entire being. He restored His physical body as He slept, He exercised, and He got fresh air and sunshine. He restored His mind (learned to relax) by finding a peaceful place of solitude, far from the customary press of the crowds—filled with curiosity-seekers, the sick, and religious leaders who opposed Him. He restored His spirit by communicating one on one with God.

As I said earlier, we are three-part beings of body, soul (mind, will, and emotions), and spirit. Like Jesus, we need restoration in all those areas. In Mark 1:35 Jesus painted a beautiful picture of how to get healthy and stay healthy.

Christ's healthy habits enabled Him to accomplish the work God set before Him. When the disciples found Him that morning and informed Him that everyone was looking for Him, Jesus felt refreshed and ready to minister again. The disciples were probably eager to walk back to the village and eat breakfast, but Jesus had much bigger plans: "Let us go into the next towns, that I may preach there also, because for this purpose I have come forth" (Mark 1:36). Then look what He did: "He went to their meeting places all through Galilee, preaching and throwing out the demons" (vv. 38–39, The Message). Sounds like Jesus had more than enough energy to fulfill God's call.

SIMPLE YET PROFOUND: WHY CAN'T YOU SLEEP?

Why can't you sleep? Here are a few factors and some suggestions for overcoming them.

Menopause, sleep apnea, and restless legs

As you age, several factors can hinder the quality and quantity of your sleep. For women, menopausal hot flashes and night sweats can interrupt it. However, recent studies indicate that menopausal women are also likely to suffer from two other age-related sleep problems: sleep apnea and restless leg syndrome (RLS). Maintaining a healthy body weight can help with sleep apnea. Your doctor may also recommend therapeutic devices to help you keep your airways open. RLS may respond to improved nutrition, vitamin and iron supplements, exercise, and removing caffeine and alcohol from your diet.

Mind over matter

Many of us also suffer from RMS—restless mind syndrome! You can sag into bed feeling *so* tired and your bed feels *so* good, yet your brain just won't stop running. One way to quiet your mind is through quiet prayer and reflection on God's Word before you retire. Another aid is trying an herbal adjunct, such as a hot cup of green tea with lemon balm. Green tea contains an amino acid, L-theanine, which has been shown to reduce physical and mental stress and helps your brain produce soothing alpha waves.

Mellow out with melatonin

Another factor, imbalanced melatonin production, can wreak havoc on your sleep cycles. Melatonin is a hormone that enables deep, healthy sleep. Older folks tend to produce less melatonin than they need at night and more during the day when it causes drowsiness. Sleeping in total darkness can help restore a balanced melatonin production schedule. Melatonin is available as a supplement; ask your doctor if he or she would recommend this.

The half-night sleep

Do you find it easy to fall asleep, only to awake a few hours later and wind up with an agonizing, sleepless second half of the night? This type of sleep pattern deprives you of the several complete sleep cycles needed to maintain health. Even a nap during the day can't make up for losing sleep at night. An ancient herb called valerian may help you get to sleep and stay asleep. Valerian increases the levels of the amino acid GABA in your system. GABA induces sleep while helping to regulate relaxation and anxiety.

Medications and illnesses

If you are taking a prescription for blood pressure or seizures, or are using antidepressants, diuretics, or stimulants (diet pills or amphetamines), you may have trouble getting a good night's sleep. Discuss this further with your doctor. Heart disease, respiratory disease, GI problems, and endocrine disease are just a few ailments that can also interfere with your sleep cycle.

Ready to learn about the third key to good health? Then get moving.

CHAPTER 3

KEY 3:
FAITH IS A MOVING
EXPERIENCE: EXERCISE!

IN JESUS'S ERA only the rich traveled by horse. The Bible refers to people occasionally traveling by boat, but typically when on land they walked. Other than riding into Jerusalem on a donkey at Passover, Jesus walked almost everywhere He went. So did His disciples. They all got their exercise—it was an inescapable part of their daily routine.

Not so in the twenty-first century. Many of us escape exercise as often as possible. We drive to work, sit at our desks all day, and then drive home and sit in front of the TV. That is a lot of sitting and not much exercise, unless we count tapping on keyboards or lifting food to our mouths as exercise. These habits run counter to my third vital key to good health: exercise.

Right now you may be grumbling, "I knew that 'E' word would show up somewhere." Well, if Jesus exercised every day, then what makes us think we should be immune from this good health habit? Only we don't *have to* exercise to get from one place to another; we *get to* for our health.

Having to do something seems negative; *getting to* do something seems positive. I like to concentrate on the positive, so I always say *get to* instead of *have to*. My kids always see that one coming. By now whenever I say, "You don't *have to* do this, you know," they quickly finish my thought with, "We know, we know, Dad. We *get to* do it."

Since you and I *get to* exercise, we should think of it as a privilege. Exercise *is* a privilege, an opportunity to reap the blessings of good health. We often tend to think of physical activity in negative terms. We look at it as an interruption to our day, one more thing to cram into our busy schedule, and something that brings pain to boot. In reality we don't pay a price for following good health habits—we pay dearly for poor health habits.

You and I don't need to end up in the hospital or confined to a room at home because we ate fat-filled meals, snacked on junk food, and never walked around the block. And with simple, small changes in our daily routines to incorporate exercise, we can do what Jesus did—walk. The average person in His day walked three to ten miles a day. Jesus Himself walked well over twenty thousand miles over the course of His ministry!

Since my mother lives in close proximity, I sometimes feel like Raymond on the hit show *Everybody Loves Raymond*. Only in my case Mom lives next door instead of across the street. Even though its nine-year-long run ended in 2005, Raymond lives on through reruns on cable stations in the United States and worldwide, plus DVD collections. Now I'm not a wise-cracking sportswriter and try not to continually evade responsibility, but like Raymond I some-times get the short end of the stick.

Mostly though it's great having Mom next door—especially since my father has gone on to heaven. Since she is retired, Mom loves to have her grandkids over to visit and keep her company. Many mornings, particularly on the weekends, one or more trek across the yard to see her.

One morning our son walked over to see Grandma, who was exercising in front of her TV, which was tuned to fitness expert Denise Austin's program. She knew Donnie would want to watch cartoons, so she told him he could have the TV as soon as she finished. Sitting there blinking sleep out of his eyes, he patiently waited for her session to end. After several minutes of watching his grandmother exercising in synch with Austin, he said with a deadpan look, "You know, Grandma, you're never going to look like her."

Mom got a big laugh out of that one! Particularly since, in her early seventies, she is in tip-top condition. One of her favorite sayings is, "If I don't move it, I'll lose it." How true. And although exercise may not restore the fresh-faced beauty or handsome physique you enjoyed in your twenties, it will go a long way toward making you feel young and trim again. My mother is living proof. She is beautiful and sharp despite her age. After all, exercisers are three to five times less likely to suffer from Alzheimer's disease.

WALKING FOR FITNESS

As I mentioned, Jesus walked well over twenty thousand miles during His time on earth. While I haven't covered twenty thousand miles yet, walking is my favorite exercise. A brisk walk of thirty to forty-five minutes, three to five days a week is almost as beneficial as jogging. Or an easier way to think of it is to do the 4:40: that is walking four days a week for forty minutes per session. You will enjoy it more than you might think, and it will make you feel terrific.

Keep in mind that you don't need to speed along fast, get your heart wildly racing, and run out of breath to make your walking count. However, it is good to do more than stroll, a habit I tend to fall into. Whenever I suggest exercising together, Susan usually declines my offer because she likes to move along briskly and get her arms swinging. "If I'm going to do this, I'm going to make it count," she tells me. Meanwhile I stroll along and tell her I'm "four-sixing it," casting all my cares on Him. Though my statements rarely convince her, at least we are exercising—even if at a different pace!

First Timothy 4:8 says, "Bodily exercise profits a little, but godliness is profitable for all things." However, in the Greek that verse literally reads, "Bodily exercise profits for a season, but spiritual exercise is profitable eternally." For what season is bodily exercise profitable? For the season that you are in your physical body here on earth! You are God's temple—His mobile home, so to speak. You only get to travel around down here for as long as your body lasts. Healthy bodies make the journey much easier.

IT'S NEVER TOO LATE

Americans love to talk about exercise, but not many of them follow through and do it. Ninety percent of the public rates exercise as essential to good health, but only 20 percent actually do it. If you are among the nonexercising majority, take heart. No matter how old you are or what kind of shape you are in, it is never too late to get moving to strengthen your body and help it last longer.

I want to recommend a great move to get you started. The best thing about it is that you can even do this while watching TV (not that I recommend you exercise in front of the TV all the time, but you have to start somewhere). During every commercial do chair lifts. Have you ever seen weight lifters do squats in a gym? This is the same principle. Stand up as soon as a commercial starts, then squat down until your back end nearly touches your chair again—but not quite. Then jump up, springing as high as you can with your hands in the air.

Chair lifts work every major muscle group and are aerobic as well. They are a simple move with complex benefits. Do chair lifts as many times as you can during commercials, aiming for a goal of two sets, and ten repetitions per set, during each commercial break. Once you hit that goal, take it to the next level by adding a can of soup in each hand for resistance.

Imagine the good shape you could be in if you had done chair lifts for every commercial you have ever watched! From now on, instead of running to the refrigerator or snacks in the pantry during commercials, do this exercise. It won't take long to notice a big difference in how you look and feel.

THE ASTONISHING BENEFITS

Exercise does wonderful things for your body. First, it releases endorphins, which are "feel-good" neurotransmitters (brain chemicals) that literally make you feel better. That's why some depression can be treated with consistent exercise. Exercise is also the number one treatment for osteoporosis—thinning of the bones—as well as hypertension (high blood pressure), insomnia (trouble sleeping), and many other ailments.

Studies show that four hours of exercise a week reduces a woman's risk of breast cancer by 60 percent! That alone makes it worth the effort for any female. In addition, exercise has been shown to reduce the risk of colon cancer, pancreatic cancer, and prostate cancer. Exercise can prevent, control, and even *reverse* adult-onset diabetes, because it reduces fat and allows insulin to start working again. With nearly

11 million people ages sixty-five or older (26.9 percent) suffering from diabetes and 1.9 million newly diagnosed cases among adults twenty or older in 2010,[1] this makes exercise well worth the effort. I can't think of one ailment that can't be addressed beneficially by exercise.

Exercise strengthens your heart muscle and increases your circulation (blood flow) too. As God's Word says, "The life of the flesh is in the blood" (Lev. 17:11). The oxygen-carrying capacity of your body increases as your blood flow increases—and that's good news because all diseases hate oxygen!

While diseases hate oxygen, your brain loves it. The more you exercise, the more oxygen reaches your brain and the better your mental state. Exercise is the one and only thing that will increase mental alertness and emotional tranquility. Best of all, other than a little sweat, it has no side effects. Doesn't it sound good to have mental clarity when you need it and also be able to relax and feel peaceful inside?

How about all those people you have heard about who had to have heart-bypass surgery? Did you know regular exercise promotes natural bypasses? Your body continually makes collateral arterials, which are "alternate routes" that blood can flow through should the main routes be blocked. Exercise is the only way to consistently increase this vital circulation. The more you exercise, the more collateral arterials your body makes. Whatever physical problem a person may have, increasing blood flow by way of consistent, moderate exercise can be a vital element of treatment.

What about migraines? If you have ever been incapacitated by one of those splitting headaches, you know all about pain and suffering. If you suffer from them, I have great news for you. Studies show that increasing your water intake and engaging in consistent, moderate exercise markedly decreases—and often completely eliminates—the incidence of migraines. That spells relief the natural way.

EXERCISE AND THE HEALTH EQUATION

Why are people who consistently exercise healthier? Exercise helps balance the health equation. Remember the health equation that I mentioned in the introduction? If not, here it is again:

Detoxification + balancing the immune system = great health

The immune system moves its contents around your body via the lymphatic system. You generally have three to five times as much lymphatic fluid in your body as you do blood. Your circulatory system has a pump (the heart) that circulates blood, but your lymphatic system does not have a pump to circulate lymphatic fluid. It is a passive system that contains one-way valves but no pump, so lymphatic or immune system fluids don't move around inside much unless *you* move.

The lymphatic fluid of a sedentary person circulates through his or her body about once a day. In someone who exercises, it circulates three or four times a day. That is a statistically significant difference and the reason that people who consistently exercise have stronger immune systems. The lymphatic fluid with its immune-boosting ingredients moves throughout their bodies more often.

Since moving your muscles moves your lymphatic fluids, move *somehow*. If all you can do because of your health issues is walk once around the block, then walk around the block! I had a friend who said all he could do was get up in the morning and walk four times around the block. I thought that was a decent start toward exercising, until he told me that after he finished, he slid the block under his bed and went back to sleep!

Don't let your avoidance of exercise keep you pinned in bed. As the Nike commercial says, "Just do it." If all you can do when you're sick is move one leg, then move that leg! Move whatever you can move to get that immune system fluid circulating.

As an added bonus, exercise also helps the body properly detoxify. Not only do you sweat out toxins, but also thirst-inducing exercise means you will tend to drink more water, the ultimate body purifier. Sweating is a fantastic way to detox, but remember that you also sweat out minerals when you work out. As you engage in an exercise program, make sure you replace the minerals you lose with a good supplement. (I will cover supplements briefly in the final chapter.)

I already mentioned that exercise releases endogenous morphines called endorphins throughout your body. Those act as your body's natural painkillers. Have you ever wondered how on earth people who start exercising and stick with it wind up *enjoying* it? Now you know. Regular exercisers experience the pleasant effects of endorphins released in their systems. In fact, when they skip it, they actually miss exercising. Wouldn't you like to be in that position? You can be if you start and stick with it.

THE "W" WORD

The infamy of the "E" word, *exercise*, is nothing compared to the infamy of the "W" word, but we might as well cover them both. Are you ready? Don't stop reading when you find out that the "W" word is *weight*. Before you panic, realize that *you are not what you weigh*. By that I mean your health is not dependent on whether you fit within the "normal" weight range for your height on those equally infamous body mass index (BMI) charts.

So often we judge ourselves by the reading on the scale, but it isn't about the numbers. What is more important is how you feel and how your energy level holds up to whatever God is calling you to do. As a physician, what you weigh right now means far less to me than what you are doing for your health on a daily basis. I recommend that you "live it" rather than "die-it." Instead of buying into every fad diet that comes down the pike and watching your weight bounce up and down like a roller coaster, start "doing the dos," particularly exercising and eating wholesome, God-made foods. Those lifestyle habits will get you to your *ideal* weight eventually and keep you there.

As we travel and teach on my Ten Keys That Cure, we meet many people who are very thin yet very unhealthy, just as I was in medical school. We meet people who, while at their perfect chart weight, are unhealthy because they aren't "doing the dos." We also meet those who are technically overweight, yet because they are starting to do the right things, they are reaping the benefits.

One of the best things anyone can do to reach his or her ideal weight is exercise. Why does it seem like the "E" word and "W" word always go together? Because exercise builds muscle. When trying to reach and maintain your ideal weight, muscle is your best friend. It is crucial to build muscle because a pound of muscle burns forty calories a day—even at rest. A pound of fat burns only a couple calories.

Muscle is much more efficient than fat. That's the good news. The bad news is that beginning at age twenty, the average person loses one pound of lean muscle mass every year for the rest of his life. Take a minute to do the math—in the decade of the twenties, the average person loses ten pounds of lean muscle mass. This means when you're at rest, your body burns four hundred fewer calories per day at thirty than it did at twenty. Go from thirty to forty years old, and that is eight hundred fewer calories a day. By fifty—and this is really scary because I'm past fifty—it's up to twelve hundred fewer calories. That's twelve hundred calories less than I could have eaten at age twenty unless I'm willing to pay a steep price.

However, keep in mind such a scary progression is not automatic; this only takes place in the body of the *average nonexerciser*. Those who remain active will keep their muscle mass from deteriorating. If you didn't want to exercise before, this fact alone should be enough to make you an exercise-wannabe. While sitting on the couch watching the electronic income reducer and flab inducer, take action. During commercials, get going on those chair lifts I talked about. While you're at it, grab a couple cans of soup to do some bicep repetitions. You will build muscle mass before you know it!

Before you pass me off as "just another exercise fanatic," remember these eloquent words from Proverbs: "He who does not use his endeavors to heal himself is brother to him who commits suicide" (Prov. 18:9, AMP). A footnote on this verse says it "squarely addresses the problem of whether one has a moral right to neglect his body by 'letting nature take its unhindered course' in illness." Heaven forbid we should neglect our bodies! Since God's Word tells us to do our part, we need to get moving. We have a moral obligation to use our endeavors to heal ourselves.

Statistics show that for every hour you exercise, you add two hours to your life. That is what I call endeavoring to heal yourself. I'll never forget mentioning this statistic at a health club where a seventy-five-year-old lady sat in the front row, wearing her jogging suit and a headband. Just back from a five-mile run, she perched on the edge of her seat, soaking up my presentation. When I mentioned this statistic, she piped up, "At that rate, I'll never die!" I still haven't done the math to figure that one out. I do know, though, that for all of us, exercise will certainly help our earth suits last longer.

SIMPLE YET PROFOUND: WORKING IN A WORKOUT

For the concluding section, I turn to words of wisdom from my better half.

Hi! Susan here. I know how difficult it can be to work in a workout. After I gave birth to our fourth child, I felt incredibly discouraged looking at the out-of-shape, baggy-eyed reflection in the mirror every morning. I had so many clothes jammed in my closet that I couldn't squeeze my post-baby fat into. Though I knew it was time to get back in shape, I wondered, "How?" Between my part-time job, caring for four children, supporting Dr. Don in his ministry, doing laundry, trying to cook healthy dinners...not to mention dinner, the dishes, and other household tasks...where exactly was it I supposed to find the time?

Well, this is where my faith came in handy. I took this issue to the Lord in prayer, and He answered. Right about that time the company I worked for offered its employees free memberships in a nearby gym and fitness club. Not only did I take them up on the offer, but I also decided I simply had to make time in my day by scheduling workouts as I would any other appointment. Then I committed to it. I never asked myself if I "feel like" exercising; I just did it.

However, even if you don't have the opportunity to visit a fitness center, you still can work activity into your daily life. Rest assured of this point: the Lord wants you healthy and will help you meet your goals.

At home I keep moving too. Here are some other ways that I work in a workout into my daily schedule.

On the phone

While stuck on hold (and who hasn't been there?) or even during a pleasant conversation with a friend, take the opportunity to stretch. Bend at the waist to stretch out the backs of your legs. Twist side to side to loosen your back. Tip your head side to side to release tension in your neck. If you can without losing track of the phone, sit down and circle your ankles, clockwise and counterclockwise.

While watching TV

Have hand weights close by so you can do reps while you watch. Curl your hands up toward your body to work the biceps. Hold weights in the center and lift with your elbows leading to work upper arms. Hold the weights interlocked behind your head and lift to work off under-the-arm flab. During commercials do ten crunches or push-ups.

Cleaning for health

I also find vacuuming and dusting make good "arm and shoulder" workouts, while picking up toys offers good opportunities for some quick squats to bend the legs. Make the most of your steps around the house by swinging your arms or taking a moment to stretch. Both are good ways to get your blood flowing, especially if you have been sitting at a computer for a long time.

Morning and night

I always try to do ten push-ups first thing in the morning and another ten just before I get into bed at night.

Proactive parking

Instead of stressing out as you try to find the closest parking space to the office or shopping center door, park at the outer edge of the parking lot so you can regularly work extra steps into your life.

Of course, putting a more formal workout into your schedule will provide even more benefits. If just getting started, find an activity you enjoy doing and then make it a priority. Since I really like classes and draw motivation from the enthusiasm that comes from group settings, I often sign up for these kind of sessions. Since I hate cycling, you won't find me in any of those spinning classes! When you choose something that you like to do, you are more likely to continue.

In addition, invite a friend to join you. You will increase the fun factor and add a measure of accountability. If you can't find a friend whose schedule meshes with yours, join a class and make some new friends!

CHAPTER 4

KEY 4:
GREAT HEALTH IN THE GREAT
OUTDOORS: BREATHE FRESH AIR

B REATHE MORE FRESH air. Sounds simple, doesn't it? Yet as I
discuss this topic with numerous audiences in my speaking
and teaching sessions, I am surprised by the large number
of people who regularly neglect to get outdoors so they can breathe
fresh air. As important as relaxation, adequate rest, and exercise, this
is fourth on my list of ten keys.

Fresh air does you a world of good. Between time spent in the
office or school, watching TV, playing video games, or surfing the
Internet, far too many people get limited exposure to nature's healthy
oxygen. Breathing fresh air can give you a stronger sense of well-
being, promote relaxation, and improve lung functions. With the
current increased migration to congested, more polluted urban areas,
finding fresh air can be a challenge. Still it is worth the effort to get
to a nearby park or river, a forest or wooded area just outside of the
city, or a hilly area where you can take a hike and fill your lungs.

Not only is breathing fresh air vital to good health, so is the
practice of deep breathing. I suppose the failure of many people to

engage in this basic discipline isn't too surprising. After all, when I started to research health and longevity, I found little emphasis on proper breathing in most of the medical literature I initially surveyed. However, after a more thorough study that helped me learn about its benefits, I implement deep breathing on a daily basis. I even schedule time for it five or six times a week during exercise routines.

This has boosted my health in a number of ways. Deep breathing brought noticeable improvements to my workouts, curtailed problems I had experienced with afternoon fatigue, and enhanced my sleep patterns. In the past I often awoke too early and had trouble falling back to sleep.

Now I am not just talking about the extra breathing that automatically occurs whenever you exercise. (The "bonus breathing" attached to consistently moving your body has merits of its own.) Instead, I am referring to taking the time to practice deep breathing as a way to promote good health. There are few things we take for granted as much as the air we breathe. Without effort or intentionality, the process of inhaling and exhaling continues from our first breath on earth to our last. Many people don't recognize that breathing represents an absolutely miraculous exchange of gases—which is responsible for perhaps the most important physiologic event sustaining life.

So let's pause momentarily, take a deep breath, and consider why and how we breathe. Doctors who specialize in the study and treatment of lung diseases routinely measure a lung function called "vital capacity." Simply defined, this is the amount of air a person is able to inhale and exhale with one giant breath. It is also a gross yet quite reliable assessment of how efficiently the lungs are functioning. The greater the vital capacity, the greater the ability the body has to take in essential oxygen and remove harmful carbon dioxide. Anything that increases vital capacity helps to keep your body well supplied with oxygen. Oxygen is the nutrient required to convert the food you eat into life-giving energy. Think of it as another simple health formula:

More oxygen = more energy

As your cells' number one nutrient, oxygen is vital to your cells every second of every day. Since all bodily functions depend on breathing, proper oxygen delivery to every cell of your body is essential to life. Conversely, some experts believe oxygen deficiency is the single greatest cause of disease.

Since it delivers needed oxygen, deep breathing relaxes muscles, helps relieve aches and pains, and fights disease in several ways. Most importantly it provides your cells with the oxygen they require for healthy functioning. Like exercise, oxygen helps move lymphatic fluid through your body. Taking a deep breath creates an inner vacuum effect, pulling lymphatic fluid throughout your immune system. Cancer, infection, and diseases of every sort hate oxygen, so gulping deep breaths of fresh air helps fight them off.

IT KEEPS GETTING BETTER

There are even more benefits to deep breathing. Besides balancing your immune system, it enhances detoxification, the other crucial part of the health equation. Deep breathing can increase your body's rate of toxic elimination by as much as fifteen times the normal rate. That's huge!

If this weren't enough, deep breathing is a fantastic technique for combating stress by helping you four-six it (casting all your cares on the Lord). Try this—breathe in for four seconds, then hold it for four seconds. Then breathe out slowly. You just relieved stress. You broke your focus off anything you were going through and took time to relax and refresh every cell in your body. You can do this anytime, anywhere.

Breathing happens automatically; you aren't even thinking about breathing as you read this material. Yet your respiratory system is part of God's marvelous design of your body that promotes good health. Use it fully as God intended, and you will reap huge health benefits. So keep breathing fresh air. It sure beats the alternative!

You should be aware that just as deep breathing is healthy, shallow breathing is not. This is primarily because it does not adequately allow the body to remove acidifying carbon dioxide. Proper breathing helps keep the pH levels in your blood balanced in an alkaline direction, which promotes healing processes. A more acidic body leans toward increasing free-radical damage—which basically means aging—as well as all of the chronic degenerative diseases that are more common as we grow older.

Another major benefit of breathing properly is that it aids in expanding lung volume. This expands your blood's oxygen-carrying capacity. The deeper you breathe, the more that the service area lining your lungs gets exposed to life-giving oxygen. After the lungs pick up this oxygen, the hemoglobin molecules found in red blood cells are immediately delivered throughout the body. Increasing oxygen to the muscles reduces fatigue and enhances energy levels.

In addition, when the brain gets more oxygen, the ability of neurons to communicate with one another is more efficient. This promotes clearer, more focused thinking. Plus, more oxygen to the heart means increased stamina, longevity, and ability to exercise. When the gastrointestinal tract receives its share of oxygen, not only does it improve digestion and absorption of nutrients, but there is also a specific, direct boost to the immune system. Since more than 70 percent of the immune system is located in or near the digestive tract, deep breathing can improve self-immunity, acting like a natural "self-vaccination."

The process of metabolism, or burning calories, requires an enormous amount of oxygen. With healthy deep breathing, the food you eat will be more efficiently converted to energy rather than stored as fat. Breathing properly can also increase thermogenesis—the rate at which you burn calories.

So how do we breathe properly? In her book *Prescription for Nutritional Healing*, longtime nutrition counselor author Phyllis Balch gives more detail about the effects of deep breathing. Here I will simply offer two brief prescriptions for enhancing your body's healing capacity through deep breathing.

First, practice the following:

1. Slowly breathe in through your nose with mouth closed to maximum lung capacity using the diaphragm. This means pulling your stomach in as much as you can when you take your deep breath.

2. Hold for a count of ten.

3. Slowly exhale through your mouth.

Do this for five minutes, three times a day, preferably in an outdoor, nonpolluted atmosphere.

For quick relaxation, try the following technique:

1. Place arms straight down along the sides of the body. As you inhale deeply, lift arms up and out as if to form a "V" shape.

2. Exhale slowly through your mouth as you bring your arms back down to your sides.

This formula combines breathing and exercise and can be done hourly to refresh and remove stress hormones. All together now, inhale deeply—all day long.

SIMPLE YET PROFOUND: GO SMOKE FREE FOR GOD

It goes without saying that the key of breathing fresh air leaves no room for smoking, which fouls your lungs as well as the environment around you. Although I want to focus on the positive things you can do for your health rather than a list of "do nots," I can't help acknowledging that many people struggle with a nicotine addiction. So I will add a quick word that I hope will help. If you are a smoker, did you know that quitting means vastly enhancing the potential of improving your health? It will literally skyrocket.

For most smokers, within two years from the time they stop 80 percent of the negative changes in their lungs will disappear. For longtime smokers over the age of fifty, this rehabilitative process may take up to four years, but they will eventually get it back. This healing aspect of quitting smoking is absolutely phenomenal! Farther down the road almost all of smoking's negative effects on your respiratory system will vanish. There is no better time to stop than today.

Now I don't want to give you the idea that breaking this (or any) bad habit is a simple matter. Still I have a suggestion for you smokers that you can implement for about seventy-nine cents. For that price you can buy a small squeeze bottle of lemon juice at the grocery store. Each and every time you crave a cigarette, put that little bottle in your mouth and give it a good squeeze. It will do a couple things: 1)

The shock will "reset" your system—literally. As your taste buds react to the lemon juice, you'll forget your nicotine urge. 2) It will provide some negative conditioning. Most people don't enjoy the taste of lemon juice—an understatement—and you will start thinking twice before contemplating another cigarette. (If you're one of those rare people who like lemon juice, then it will at least provide a pleasant diversion.) Try the lemon juice method and see what happens.

Kicking the nicotine habit will save you money and your health, not to mention the health of those around you. Consider the nasty effects of secondhand smoke, which causes an estimated 46,000 premature deaths from heart disease each year among nonsmokers[1] and increases nonsmokers' risk of developing lung cancer by 20 to 30 percent and heart disease by 25 to 30 percent. Conditions among children attributed to secondhand smoke are sudden infant death syndrome, respiratory infections, asthma attacks, ear infections, and chronic cough.[2]

"Secondhand smoke is similar to the mainstream smoke inhaled by the smoker in that it is a complex mixture containing many chemicals (including formaldehyde, cyanide, carbon monoxide, ammonia, and nicotine), many of which are known carcinogens," says a major report from the US Surgeon General's office. "Exposure to secondhand smoke causes excess deaths in the U.S. population from lung cancer and cardiac related illnesses...exposure to secondhand smoke remains an alarming public health hazard. Approximately 60 percent of nonsmokers in the United States have biological evidence of exposure to secondhand smoke."[3]

Best of all, kicking the nicotine habit will enable you to breathe fresh air deeply and benefit from it fully, as God intended.

CHAPTER 5

KEY 5:
GREAT HEALTH IN THE GREAT
OUTDOORS: SUNSHINE

YOU CAN'T BUY sunshine by the bottle. Nature's tonic for the soul is free. Sunshine is good for many things that ail you—and is my fifth key for healthy living.

I love basking in the sunshine. It makes me and millions of other folks feel better.

Many of you may be surprised that sunshine is one of my Ten Keys That Cure. Given the typical overreaction that seems to greet the latest health or diet proclamation (remember when everyone went nuts about eating oat bran?), millions today seem to fear one of the greatest blessings God ever created.

One reason is because many doctors (especially dermatologists) are warning their patients about the dangers of sun exposure. However, they should emphasize the dangers of *overexposure*. The sun is something to be enjoyed not feared. Sun is an excellent source of vitamin D, which helps control calcium and phosphorus levels and plays a role in cell growth, the immune system, and reducing inflammation in the body.

In addition it is difficult to get adequate vitamin D from food alone, according to Elisabetta Politi, nutrition director at the Duke Diet and Fitness Center. While such fatty fish as salmon and fortified dairy products, juices, and cereals are good sources, she says you would have to eat them every day to get the daily requirements. And Politi says, "Mushrooms are one of the only D-rich vegetables."[1]

If this hasn't convinced you of the benefits of sunshine, it is worth noting that Politi says about 50 percent of Americans don't get enough vitamin D. That is one reason she believes in taking a multivitamin with 800 to 1,000 international units of vitamin D. Supplements can help add to your sun intake. Why is this vitamin so important? Because low levels have been linked to osteoporosis, fibromyalgia, colon cancer, gingivitis (inflammation of the gums), and such immune system disorders as rheumatoid arthritis, lupus, and type 1 diabetes.

AFFECTED BY THE SEASONS

Lack of sun can cause more than physical disease; it can affect your mental outlook as well. In 1984 officials at the National Institute of Mental Health came up with a name for the winter blues: seasonal affective disorder (SAD). Among its symptoms are depression, increased appetite with weight gain (weight loss is more common with other forms of depression), diminished energy, and loss of interest in work or other activities.

After living through some of these symptoms during the freezing, snowy winters, I can assure you SAD is for real. For many long, cloudy Michigan winters I just did not feel right. I noticed that when business took me south during this season, I felt much better. Finally, I realized that the authorities who had named this commonly winter-linked disorder were on to something. It wasn't just a simple matter of "bucking up," reading a good book, or socializing a little more.

When I realized these symptoms were real and could be addressed, I implemented two simple changes that proved to be life-changing for my family and me:

- **First, I replaced our conventional light bulbs at home with full-spectrum, natural bulbs.** Full-spectrum bulbs made a noticeable impact in our home, especially next to the chair where I do most of my reading. This gave me immediate benefits, particularly when I spent two hours a day or more in their light. They are money-savers too, using far less wattage to produce energy. This is economical and good for the environment.

- **Although this may strike some as a bit controversial, I started using a special tanning bed.** As with people who go overboard and declare everyone should avoid the sun, you can go to extremes and label me a nut for recommending a tanning bed. However, it is significant to realize that I used one for only about five minutes a week. Besides helping me avoid SAD symptoms, this experience had a pleasant (and surprising) side effect. After several sessions, I found that the mild eczema and psoriasis on the end of my thumb and two fingers noticeably improved.

Certainly I am not recommending overuse of a tanning booth. The dangers are obvious—but then so is spending all day in the sun.

If you struggle with seasonal depression, a skin condition, or moodiness during times of limited sun exposure, try some of these simple things and see what happens. If nothing else, you will end up with a healthy glow and look a little better. Remember the healthiest skin is slightly tanned, well-hydrated skin. So get into the light—and drink more of what you're made of: fresh purified water (more about that in the tenth key).

LIMITING EXPOSURE

Granted, you need to limit your exposure to the sun. Nobody wants to suffer horrendous sunburn or its ill effects on health and personal comfort. However, staying completely away from the sun is even worse for you than getting exposure in small doses. Avoiding the sun or lavishing liberal amounts of sunscreen on your body every time you step outside is not good for you.

Sunshine is vital to the process of converting cholesterol in your skin into vitamin D, which promotes strong bones. The bones also happen to be where the immune system's cells are formed. No wonder people long to step out into the sunshine when they see it, and even sing about it. So go ahead—a little sunshine every day is good for you!

In fact, a recent study shows that as one of the best sources of vitamin D, exposure to sunshine can offer protection from other cancers, osteoporosis, rickets, and diabetes. Scientists at Brookhaven National Laboratory and Norway's Institute for Cancer Research say the health benefits from the sun are far greater than the risk of skin cancer. Because they get more sun, people from the earth's southern latitudes are significantly less likely to die from such internal cancers as colon, lung, breast, and prostate. The lead researcher says while doubling sun exposure could increase skin cancer deaths, such a step would decrease the rate of death from other cancers by a factor of ten.[2]

The question is, though, how much exposure to the sun is good? From a practical perspective, to manufacture adequate amounts of vitamin D you need to get out without sunscreen or while wearing long sleeves for twenty minutes, at least three times a week. If your skin is dark or if you are past the age of sixty-five, even more sunshine is required because your production of vitamin D is lower. In this case you want to soak up forty minutes of sunshine at least three times a week.

Of course you would be wise to avoid sunburn by working your way up gradually to that exposure. For example, you could choose Mondays, Wednesdays, and Fridays as your sun days, starting with five minutes of exposure that first Monday. On Wednesday double the time and on Friday go for fifteen minutes. In the following weeks continue adding five minutes to your exposure each time until you have worked your way up to forty minutes per day.

Something I always do when going out in the sun is keeping skin properly hydrated, internally and externally. I do this by making sure I drink adequate fluids (eight to twelve glasses of water a day) and by using natural skin moisturizing lotions. I apply these especially after a shower, when it is easiest to trap some of the moisture in the skin. Properly hydrated skin makes for healthy skin.

Sunshine is also intimately related to your wake-sleep cycle. The rising and falling of the sun sets your circadian rhythm—your biological clock (not in the reproductive sense, but in the body's daily functioning). If you never see the light of day, it will leave you feeling like you stepped into a time warp. As a result it will hinder your natural sense timing. Just ask someone who has worked third shift for an extended period of time.

The way we live in modern times, it is no wonder so many people complain about the aforementioned seasonal affective disorder. Never feeling the sun's warm rays or seeing its cheerful light is enough to make anyone feel gloomy and deprived. Even sitting near a window and letting sunlight hit your eyes is good for you. This light travels through your pupils into your retina and gets picked up by your brain, where the impulses go to your pineal gland. The master gland that regulates many of your body's other glands, the pineal is regulated by light and darkness. It secretes melatonin, a hormone linked to strengthening your immune system and setting your circadian rhythm.

God meant for us to enjoy the magnificent sun. As Solomon wrote, "Truly the light is sweet, and it is pleasant for the eyes to behold the sun" (Eccles. 11:7). The sun is pleasant, and it is good for you in moderation.

SIMPLE YET PROFOUND: BROCCOLI FOR SUNSCREEN?

The more I learn about commercial sunscreens, the more I want to warn my patients about the dangers of overusing them. For one, sunshine is good for you. As I said earlier, twenty minutes in the sun on a summer's day provides most people with all the vitamin D they need.

Yet as you step into the sun, be wary of the modern mania of slathering sunscreen all over the body. Scientists have raised concerns about certain chemicals in sunscreens. These are substances with strange-sounding names that mystify most people. Things such as diethanolamine (DEA), triethanolamine (TEA), padimate-o, octyl dimethyl PABA, benzophenone, oxybenzone, homosalate, octylmethoxycinnamate (octinoxate), salicylates, and parabens. The main thing you need to know about them: some are known carcinogens (cancer causers), and others attach to hormone receptors, which can mimic or block healthy hormone balance.

Because of the hazards of sunscreens, US researchers are working on a new, safer form of protection from the sun's ultraviolet radiation, a sunscreen made from extracts of broccoli sprouts (no, I'm not making this up). A team of scientists from Johns Hopkins University reported in the *Proceedings of the National Academy of Sciences* that topical application of this substance markedly reduced radiation in extract-treated skin of human volunteers and parallel evidence in mice.[3]

The significance of such a sunscreen alternative is the demand for protection from King Sol as the incidence of skin cancer has risen dramatically amid higher exposure of aging populations. The most common of all cancers, it accounts for nearly half of all cancers in the United States—more than two million cases of non-melanoma skin cancers occur annually, according to the American Cancer Society.[4]

Investigator Paul Talalay, MD, says this veggie-derived extract is not a sunscreen. Unlike sunscreens, it does not absorb ultraviolent light and prevent it from entering the skin. Instead, it works inside cells by boosting the production of a network of protective enzymes that defend against radiation damage. The effect lasts for several days, even after the extract is no longer present on or in the skin.

"Treatment with this broccoli sprout extract might be another protective measure that alleviates the skin damage caused by UV radiation and thereby decreases our long-term risk of developing cancer," says Dr. Talalay.[5]

Personally, I like wearing my broccoli on the inside. My family loves chomping on it raw to get all the wonderful nutrients that God created. Meanwhile, we get outdoors for fresh air and sunshine! I hope you will too. Don't let fear of too much sunshine cause you to overreact and camp inside or wrap yourself like a mummy when you step out the door, thereby negating its positive effects. Sunshine is good for you!

EAT, DRINK, AND BE HEALTHY!

At this point, we've made it through the first five of my Ten Keys That Cure. To quickly review: 1) learn to relax, 2) get to bed on time, 3) exercise, 4) breath fresh air, and 5) enjoy sunshine. Nothing impossible so far. Now don't you feel better knowing more about these simple steps to promoting good health?

We've seen in Mark 1:35 that Jesus used these five keys. And Ephesians 5:1 tells us we're to "be imitators of God [copy Him and follow His example]" (AMP). We need to act like Jesus in regard to our health by "doing the dos" I discussed earlier.

Next we will cover the last five keys, which have to do with what we eat and drink. Our food choices are crucial to our health. We not only need to eat and drink, but we also need to choose those substances wisely if we expect to attain good health. What food and drink choices should we make when we have an opportunity to choose? What did God intend for us to eat? Why is it true that "you are what you *ate*"? Let's move on to find the answers.

CHAPTER 6

KEY 6:
BRING FORTH FRUIT

E ATING FRUITS AND vegetables represents an excellent method. They keep us connected to the dirt—or more accurately, to the dust—from which we are made. Genesis 2:7 says, "And the LORD God formed man of the dust of the ground, and breathed into his nostrils the breath of life; and man became a living being." The original Hebrew reads "man became another speaking spirit." At the moment God breathed His breath into Adam's nostrils, God's kind of spirit life came alive in the human body.

Now to stay strong we need to stay connected to where we came from. Spiritually we need to stay connected to our Source, our Creator. We do that by daily prayer and continual reading and study of His Word. His Word is life and health to us. Those who stay connected to Him stay spiritually strong.

The same is true physically. We need to stay connected to our source. Note that Genesis 2:7 says God "formed man." *To form* is different than *to create*. God created the heavens and earth by making something that didn't exist before. When it came to humankind, though, God *formed* man. That means He took something that He had already created, the dust, and molded it into the shape of a man.

Genesis 3:19 says, "You were made from dust, and to the dust you will return" (NLT). In the meantime we will remain healthiest if we stay connected to the source of our physical makeup. We do that by eating what Susan and I call "God-made" foods. These are the foods God caused to spring up from the earth. This divine nutrition principle is so important that God mentions it in the first chapter of the Bible. When God caused the earth to bring forth plants, He said, "Behold, I have given you every herb bearing seed, which is upon the face of all the earth, and every tree, in the which is the fruit of a tree yielding seed; to you it shall be for meat [or food]" (Gen. 1:29, KJV).

"Herb-bearing seeds" and "fruit-yielding trees" refer to fruits, vegetables, and whole grains (which I will discuss later). God designed our bodies to function best on these God-made foods, not on man-made foods. When you plant a seed in rich soil, that seed will reorganize the soil's nutrients and grow into a sprout before maturing into a food-producing plant. When you come along and eat the food that seed produced, you eat reorganized dirt and reorganize it into fuel for your body. That process keeps you connected to your physical source. (If an animal comes along and beats you to the produce, you can eat the animal and still derive the benefit of staying connected to where you came from.)

In essence, when you consider the dust God formed us from and the produce we eat, we are all reorganized dirt. Don't worry, though; that doesn't make us dirtbags. In fact I like to compliment my friends by saying, "I love the way you reorganize dirt." When you are aware of the importance of literally remaking your physical body with the powerful, essential nutrients found in God-made real foods, you can expect to stay really healthy.

CHOOSE WISELY

Do you realize that the average person's food choices include an annual consumption of 750 doughnuts? That is more than two per day! Add to that 60 pounds of cakes or cookies, 23 gallons of ice cream, 22 pounds of candy, 90 pounds of fat, 365 servings of soda pop, and it is small wonder our nation struggles so mightily with obesity. First Corinthians 6:19 says that our bodies are the temples of the Holy Spirit. However, if some of us don't change what we ingest, we are going to change our small temples into large cathedrals!

Choosing to go the world's way means reaping the world's results. Because of poor food choices—downright gluttonous ones in most cases—the average American these days is both overweight and undernourished. That is nothing short of amazing in the most agriculturally productive nation in the history of the world. Every day here in the United States we produce enough food to feed ourselves while throwing away enough to feed another fifty million people! Yet the way we process most of that food robs it—and therefore us—of almost all nutrition.

I call it the "great nutrition robbery." We are depriving ourselves of the essential nutrients we need and paying dearly for it in the process. In Isaiah 55:2 God asks, "Why do you spend money for what is not bread, and your wages for what does not satisfy?" Another verse appropriately asks why we spend money on "deceitful meat" (Prov. 23:3, kjv). Indeed, why spend our hard-earned money this way? That *is* a good question!

God continues in Isaiah 55:2, "Listen carefully to Me, and eat what is good, and let your soul delight itself in abundance." This is what we need to do, but our culture is speeding rapidly in the wrong direction by processing nutrition out of our foods. Along the way we also add unhealthy and unnecessary calories. Besides huge amounts of excess sugar, our foods are laced with man-made additives. More than 2,800 FDA-approved food additives are on the market—and will wind on your pantry shelves if you're not careful when you fill your grocery cart.

FOLLOW THE OWNER'S MANUAL

When an engineer designs something complex, such as a car or computer, and you purchase it, you receive an owner's manual that helps you care for the product. If you follow the care and maintenance plan laid out in the owner's manual, you generally get long life out of your purchase. However, if you decide you are smarter than the product's creator and ignore the instructions in the owner's manual, you are likely to encounter problems. Without proper care, the product is prone to malfunction and will eventually break down.

Your car won't run smoothly if you never change the oil. Your computer will crash if you never update the virus protection. Likewise your body will break down if you don't feed it the foods it needs to maintain good health. As I have said before, your body is your most important earthly possession. Doesn't it make sense to put into practice what you read in your body's owner's manual?

I consider God's Word the owner's manual for the human body. Written by the Engineer who formed us, it gives us detailed care and maintenance instructions for body, soul (mind, will, and emotions), and spirit. Following the Bible's instructions about how to care for ourselves and each other simply makes good sense—as much sense as paying attention to a car manual.

For example, God's Word tells us to four-six it and cast all our cares on Him (Phil. 4:6). I know I am stronger spiritually when I do this. We were not created to be "care takers" but "care casters," according to 1 Peter 5:7. We are instructed to cast the whole of our care upon Him, our Maker. It also tells us that we are to have the mind of Christ (1 Cor. 2:16) and that God has given us a sound mind (2 Tim. 1:7). My mind works more clearly and my emotions are more stable when I follow God's principles.

Regarding physical maintenance, Jesus modeled my first five keys in Mark 1:35. Also, God specifically told us what to eat in Genesis 1:29. Many other Scriptures refer to food, but that verse is our designer's first mention of what we are to eat. You've perhaps already heard of the Genesis diet. Genesis 1:29 is the foundation on which that nutritional plan is built. It is a strong foundation for physical health!

Susan and I make sure that about 50 percent of our family's food intake comes from the fruits and vegetables God ordained for us to eat. You may be thinking, "That's a lot of tomatoes and cucumbers, and I'm not fond of either!" Many people feel that way. On our travels we have met numerous people who either love fruit and hate vegetables or hate fruit and love vegetables. In any case it helps to remember God loves variety. He created a seemingly endless variety of plants for us to discover and explore. Fruits and vegetables come in every shape, size, color, and taste. When was the last time you explored the taste of a new fruit or vegetable or tried a new way of preparing one you thought you didn't like?

BANANAS AND MORE

Fruit is a nutritious food that promotes all-around health. Whether in a classroom full of school children, an adult health and healing class at church, or at a seminar as a guest speaker, I always sing to my students about fruit. Sometimes they think I'm fruity, especially when I sing this verse of "Dr. Don's Be Healthy Song":

> Apples, oranges, bananas,
> Bright colors you can see,
> These are the keys to nutrition,
> Your body will agree.

Fruits are attractive because they are often brightly colored. The depth of color to a fruit (or vegetable) roughly indicates how nutrient rich it is—the brighter, the better! Fruits usually taste sweet too, meaning they are the kinds of sweets you can enjoy! Jesus did. Look at Mark 11:12: "Now the next day, when they had come out from Bethany, He was hungry. And seeing from afar a fig tree having leaves, He went to see if perhaps He would find something on it."

When Jesus was hungry, He looked for fruit such as figs. Have you tasted them? (Not Fig Newtons—I mean the real thing!) Figs are a seed pod. Research has shown that their seeds contain powerful minerals that fight cancer and all manner of disease. Their nutrients also help keep your circulatory system clean and strengthen your immune system.

Bananas are excellent because they most closely parallel the body's mineral content. When you eat a banana, you are eating the elements that compose the human body. Just about everything you need mineral-wise is conveniently packaged inside that banana peel, so make it a habit to peel back a banana every day. (Make sure to properly dispose of the wrapper, though, or your health might slip away.)

To get our kids excited about eating fruit, we get excited. We say, "Guess what we have! You won't believe this—we have *blueberries* and *watermelon*!" The kids get all excited and start shouting because they think watermelon and blueberries signal a party. Habits are as much caught as taught, so if you get excited about eating fruit, so will your kids. Kids basically do as you do, not as you say. Set the example and eat it with enthusiasm.

After all, Philippians 2:12 advises that we use "enthusiasm" in working out our salvation (AMP). *Enthusiasm* literally means "in *theos*," or God in you. Imagine that—God in you—and it should certainly keep you motivated. We all should enjoy fully working out God's plan with His tasty, naturally sweetened, powerhouse fruits! This is why we have been having watermelon-and-blueberry parties since our kids were small. There is nothing like bringing a huge, green watermelon home from the store on a hot summer day! Not to mention watermelon is a natural diuretic, helping you meet the recommended daily water intake of eight to twelve glasses.

We also enjoy eating cherries. Michigan, where we live, is famous for its production of sweet black cherries. Cherry festival time is a real celebration. Did you know cherries are especially effective in combating arthritis and gout? Cranberries are another great fruit. They're well known for their ability to combat kidney and bladder infections because of their antimicrobial activity and high vitamin C content.

Susan and the children love to put these and other fruits in cereal or in oatmeal with a touch of real maple syrup and a dash of cinnamon. Susan also tops whole-grain pancakes and waffles with fruit and real maple syrup—breakfast doesn't get any more healthy or delicious!

Another fruit my wife loves is grapefruit, although people taking cholesterol medications need to check to see whether they should avoid this form of citrus. Susan gets more excited about finding just the right color pink grapefruit than most people get over uncovering a perfectly cooked steak. It doesn't hurt that there is no fat in grapefruit—Susan can eat all she wants! She doesn't have to dig out the seeds, either. Grapefruit seeds, which so many people meticulously avoid, can and should be eaten. They contain powerful infection fighters. When it comes to cardiovascular health, grapefruits are champions. They protect arteries and balance your blood cholesterol levels, benefits likely stemming from their high fiber and high vitamin C content.

Besides grapefruit, would you believe that a kind of wonder fruit is being grown and brought to market right now that does several things for your health simultaneously? It is an excellent source of fiber (always important), and beyond that combats intestinal infections, inflammation, diarrhea, and an overly acidic stomach. More than half of your immune system is associated with your gastrointestinal tract; I always say that the road to health is paved with good intestines. This is one fruit that is excellent for good intestines.

This wonder fruit also excels at helping the body detoxify and fight viral infections. It has been shown to lower blood cholesterol and blood pressure and stabilize blood sugar. Don't you want to consume this amazing fruit every day? This well-known saying assures you that is a good idea: "An apple a day keeps the doctor away." The wonder fruit is God's magnificent creation, the apple.

The only way to find out if that saying is true is to start eating an apple a day today. (I personally believe two apples a day can keep the doctor away for twice as long.) As with the grapefruit, don't throw out the apple seeds, the skin, or the core. Did you ever see a horse spit out any part of an apple? There's a reason why another saying goes "He's as healthy as a horse." Horses eat the whole apple, and so should you.

While you may have heard that apple seeds are toxic, this is not a concern. Although they do contain trace amounts of cyanide, your normal, healthy cells contain an enzyme that renders this cyanide inactive. Interestingly cancer cells do not contain this important enzyme, so chewing apple seeds can actually help your body kill cancer cells while not harming normal cells. I call this God's chemotherapy!

EVERYTHING IN MODERATION

Although some would wish it were true, you *do not* have to bathe healthy foods in chocolate to make them palatable, even though that works. But only in moderation (everything in moderation, as the wise saying goes). Your perspective is what counts when it comes to foods such as chocolate and other so-called "sinful" treats. Are they sinful or not? Check the owner's manual. Proverbs says, "The good man eats to live, while the evil man lives to eat" (Prov. 13:25, TLB). Do you see a difference between the two? Clearly we shouldn't be obsessed with food, especially unhealthy food that replaces good nutrition and robs us of good health.

On the other hand (and you chocoholics will be glad to know there's another hand), insisting that the *only* reason we should eat is to fuel our bodies is like saying the *only* purpose for sex is procreation. Neither is true. God wants you to *enjoy* food (not to mention sex with your spouse). In the Bible food is often linked with celebrations. God's people liked to celebrate. The Old and New Testaments are full of feasting—religious feasts, wedding feasts, and dinners for Jesus at rich tax collectors' houses.

Trust me, in ancient times the Israelites ate more than leeks and onions. You can eat anything *in moderation*. As Philippians 4:5 (KJV) says, "Let your moderation be known unto all men." Susan and I teach that the food choices that *typically* characterize make the difference and that enjoying an occasional, delicious treat is not wrong.

Despite this message, some people who attend our seminars still look at us as "killjoys." At break time or when we go out to eat with them, they are afraid to eat much more than lettuce and celery sticks. If only they knew what happens on my birthday! Every year my mom makes her special-recipe chocolate cupcakes for me. Though I am *typically* characterized by healthy food choices, when my birthday comes around, health takes a holiday.

If you hear nothing else I say, let me say it again: *indulging in an occasional treat is not a problem.* Indulging in a gluttonous lifestyle is, which is why Solomon warned that you should "put a knife to your throat if you are given to gluttony" (Prov. 23:2, NIV). Gluttony is a serious issue, though most people don't think about it in those terms. They rationalize their actions with the excuse, "I'm just a junk-food junkie." Ironically, *junkie* is a more apt term than they realize. Millions of Americans don't die of old age because they dig their own graves with a knife and fork. People who are quick to condemn alcoholism and illicit drug use don't even bat an eye as they consume copious amounts of greasy, fat-filled food.

Our way of death is directly related to our way of life. My father consumed a huge number of unhealthy and unnecessary calories from junk food. At the age of fifty-six, Dad weighed 289 pounds. Not surprisingly, he blew out his aorta. God blessed him with a miracle—a skilled surgeon who repaired it. Instead of needing the usual forty units of blood during the operation, Dad needed only two. Amazed, the non-Christian surgeon commented, "We got a heavenly consult on this one!"

Dad then got serious about "doing the dos" for a while and shrank back to 200 pounds. However, his poor health habits still had a death grip on him, and he soon shot back up to 289. By then it was too late. He couldn't ward off the terrible results of self-neglect, and his heart gave out.

Besides junk food, Dad loved fried foods and used butter like frosting. Since he and Mom lived next door, I used to walk over, raid the cupboards, grab his sweet treats, and put salads in their place. Susan can tell you how furious he got, but I wanted him around to see his grandchildren grow up! However, he got to see only our sons. Our daughters won't get to meet him until we join him in heaven. I know Dad is happy up there, but down here *we* miss him. Mom misses him too. This is so sad because it didn't have to be that way.

In my younger years I certainly took after him. In the morning I would plunk a cinnamon pastry in the toaster, then after it popped, load up the backside with butter and pour a glass of soda to go with it. (I wanted caffeine, but back then I didn't like coffee.) After this unhealthy breakfast, lunch typically consisted of a burger and fries. Dinner wasn't any better. Ironically, despite a rail-thin physique, food was always on my mind—and plate. I enjoyed fast, convenient junk that satisfied my unhealthy cravings. Susan lived the same way and developed anemia in high school because of improper eating habits. The greater her vitamin and mineral deficiency, the more she craved the wrong foods.

When an animal has abnormal cravings for unhealthy substances, veterinarians call it "pica." Some horses with pica start cribbing— chewing on the wooden frames of their stalls. Obviously that is not good for them. Nor does it resolve their pica issues. And it makes their health worse.

This is how it is with some cycles humans fall into. Take what happens with chromium, an important trace mineral. You don't need a lot, but if you're not getting it, you feel bad. Chromium has many benefits: it builds muscle, helps burn fat, lowers cholesterol, balances blood sugar, and wards off mood fluctuations. When you lack chromium, you crave sweets. Yet if you eat sweets, they further deplete your body's chromium supply. The less chromium you get, the more you crave sweets. The more sweets you eat, the less chromium you have. And so the cycle goes.

It can be hard to get off that kind of merry-go-round, but until you give your body the nutritious foods it needs, you will suffer from such cycles. Pay attention to this verse of "Dr. Don's Be Healthy Song" and you will do better.

> Too much sugar will rob you
> Of minerals and vitamins.
> Sweet foods make fat—can you imagine that?
> So don't eat much of them!

By the way, sweet foods do more than make you fat and cause imbalances such as the chromium cycle. They also cause your moods to fluctuate, promoting unwelcome behaviors. You have likely heard that excess sugar causes hyperactivity in children. If you doubt it, consider a 2002 study done with prison inmates. Researchers supplemented the diets of half the inmates studied with vitamins and minerals while all of the inmates were allowed to continue their typical diet of primarily processed foods and beverages. In the supplemented group, unruly and violent behaviors markedly decreased while the violence of the group without nutritional supplements did not.[1]

The reason behind the results lies in the human brain's extreme sensitivity to any decrease in thiamin, or vitamin B_1. The excess sugar in processed foods causes the brain's level of thiamin to greatly decrease. As you might have guessed, the level of thiamin directly affects a person's inhibitory response to stimuli. In other words, when your thiamin level drops, so does your ability to say no to impulsive or improper behaviors. Without enough vitamin B_1, the brain loses its ability to manufacture certain inhibitory proteins, which are proteins that keep you from doing things you know you should not do. Simply put, you lose your inhibitions, and poor behavior becomes the rule.

As the study showed, poor decision making and poor behavior can be directly related to nutrition. When you eat nutritious foods, you increase not only your physical health but also your mental and emotional health.

SIMPLE YET PROFOUND: HOW SUSAN GETS MORE FRUIT INTO OUR DAY

Knowing you should get more fresh fruit into your daily diet is one thing. Making it happen is quite another. Our eating habits have been with us all of our lives, which makes them even harder to change. In addition, our fast-paced, twenty-first-century schedules make it easy to fall into the junk-food, fast-food, convenience-food trap. How can you keep the time crunch and its attending bad habits from sabotaging your health?

Buy it

Buy plenty of fresh fruits and vegetables so they are always on hand. Stock up with fresh apples, oranges, grapefruit, and bananas (organic if possible!). These are available year-round at your grocery store. In season, include blueberries, strawberries, and melons. When you get home from the store, rinse, slice, and store your fruit so it is easily accessible. Try setting some out in a bowl on the table or counter as an eye-catching reminder of fruit's benefits.

Snack on it

Now that you're stocked up on fresh fruit, clear out the junk food. Then, when the next snack attack hits you, you will be more likely to grab a piece of fruit instead of a cookie, chips, or some other over-processed, undernourishing snack food.

Add it to water

A squeeze of a lemon, lime, or strawberry can jazz up your glass of water, provide you fruit-based nutrition, and help you break the soda pop habit.

Cook with it

Try adding fresh blueberries to oatmeal. Top pancakes with strawberries and bananas or fill them with grated apple. Add kiwi cubes, apple slices, grapes, or dried cherries and cranberries to tossed salads.

Shake it up

Add fresh or frozen berries to plain yogurt or a protein shake.

Bring it along

When you leave the house, bring a small cooler of fruit along for the ride. Make fruit and veggies your first pick when packing lunches.

Midnight snack it

Have fruit on hand for those nights when you wake up and can't get back to sleep. It is much easier to digest than processed junk and won't interfere with resuming a good night's sleep.

Now read on for a look at the health benefits of veggies.

CHAPTER 7

KEY 7:
VEGETABLES KEEP YOU FRESH

I F YOU REMEMBER my little ditty from the last chapter, this is the one I sing after the fruit verse:

Broccoli, cabbage, and carrots
Will go to work for you;
They fight cancer and aging
And make you feel good too.

Vegetables are incredible! Jesus ate them. Some versions of Matthew 12:1 relate an incident where Jesus and His disciples were walking through a field of corn on the Sabbath. Since they were hungry, they plucked some ears and ate them. (Some versions say the field contained grain or wheat—those are healthy too. I will look at them next.) Jesus and His followers were right in thinking that eating raw corn was a good way to satisfy their hunger. You might think, "Raw corn? Who would eat that?" Well, raw corn is one of the healthiest foods for your gastrointestinal tract. Try it sometime.

We are raising our kids to follow Jesus in their eating habits. One day Susan took our hungry horde to the grocery store (always a questionable move). In the produce section one grabbed a cucumber and another an ear of corn. From their perch in the back of the grocery cart they ate their vegetables. Susan says it was cute, but the strange looks others shot her way bothered her. The kids were getting strange looks too, because they were obviously enjoying their choices.

We learned that the easiest way to get our family to eat vegetables every day is to make veggies attractive and available. My mom is good at cutting up veggies and setting them out for snacking at her house, where our kids regularly traipse through. If you cut up celery, carrots, cherry tomatoes, broccoli, and cauliflower into small, snack-sized pieces, you will be amazed at how fast those veggies will disappear from the tray you leave sitting on the counter.

Susan likes to start the day by letting the kids create fruit and vegetable faces on paper plates. The faces change every day, depending on what's in the refrigerator. This is a great way to expose the kids to different foods. Cucumber eyes look great with carrot pupils. Green or red peppers make perfect mouths. Celery works well for the ears, and an almond or walnut makes a nice nose. Don't forget to slice some fruit in thin strands or sticks for the hair!

Vegetables provide nutrients you can't get anywhere else. Did you know cabbage is the only known food source of vitamin Q? Did you even know there was a vitamin Q? It may be more familiar as the popular supplement coenzyme Q_{10} (or CoQ_{10}), which has such benefits as cancer prevention, promoting cardiovascular health, and providing energy. Eat your cabbage, and you will get it. Cabbage, broccoli, carrots, brussels sprouts, and cauliflower are some of the cruciferous vegetables that are major cancer fighters. They are full of vitamins A, C, and E, the trace mineral selenium, antioxidants, and antiaging nutrients. What a lineup! You can't achieve good health without them.

In fact, if you compare the one-fourth of the US population who eat the *fewest* fruits and vegetables with the one-fourth who eat the *most* fruits and vegetables, you will discover that the fourth who eat the fewest have a cancer rate twice as high as those who eat the most. Double the cancer rate! That is a shocking statistic!

Which group would you prefer to be in? I don't know about you, but I know which group my family and I prefer to join. We eat our fruits and vegetables every day. And we enjoy them! So will you if you use a little creativity and retrain your palate. As a result you will be much healthier too.

Anyone who had heard a gross-out joke about the effect of beans realizes that this "musical fruit" and bowel function go together. One time as I taught about normal bowel functions during a seminar at a church, I explained that the bowel is a temporary waste tank. The average American walks around with two to ten extra meals in his or her abdomen because of failing to cleanse the colon. This means toxic wastes sit in the body much longer than they should. I explained how important it is to have a bowel movement every day and that increasing water and fiber intake help empty the bowel more efficiently. The pastor mulled that over for a few seconds, jumped up, and said to his congregation, "I think what Dr. Don is trying to tell us is that it's not what you don't do that counts; it's what you doo-doo!"

Though a little graphic, his remark was essentially on target. If you don't experience daily bowel movements, your detoxification system isn't working properly. The Chinese have known this for a long time. A doctor who trained in China told me that one friendly greeting there literally means, "Have you had your bowel movement today?" By the way, in America I wouldn't try that one on the next person you meet.

Still, daily bowel function is a vital indicator of good health.

People who eat enough fruits, vegetables, and whole grains generally have an intestinal transit time of twenty-four hours or less. In other words, food enters their body, and within twenty-four hours the waste products from that food exit the body. This is a healthy pattern. Fiber, the major structural component of God-made foods, is the primary internal component needed for that kind of regularity.

Want a leading dietetic indicator of the danger of high-fat, high-sugar, low-fiber eating habits? People who follow this kind of unhealthy plan typically have an intestinal transit time of *seven days*. And, as odd as this may sound, they also have bowel movements that sink to the bottom of the toilet bowl. "Sinkers" indicate an unhealthy diet and "floaters" one that is more nutritious. Nutritious diets contain adequate fiber, which is activated by adequate amounts of water to do its work in the intestines. People who take in enough fiber and water have bowel movements that are larger and less dense. Thus, their waste products float.

If you want to check your general intestinal health, eat some corn and then watch for it. While this may sound a tad embarrassing, it is one way to check and see if you are getting enough fiber. Determine your transit time by eating some corn and then observe how long it takes to work its way through your intestinal system. If more than a day, increase your fiber intake accordingly.

Fiber detoxifies you, fills you up instead of out, and acts as an internal broom to sweep away the accumulation of bad fats and their toxins. Getting the fiber you need will change your life, and possibly your future. Illnesses such as colitis, diverticulosis, diverticulitis, and colon cancer are completely preventable—and in many cases reversible—with proper attention to fiber and water intake.

TRAINING YOUR KIDS
TO EAT VEGGIES

"Train up a child in the way he should go," says Proverbs 22:6, "and when he is old he will not depart from it." Train your kids early to choose God-made foods instead of man-made foods. Then, when they are older, they will be accustomed to making good food choices. And they will have you to thank for their good health.

In the Hebrew, to "train up a child in the way he should go" literally means to "touch the palate" of the child. Jewish mothers used to touch the upper roof of their children's mouths with whatever foods they wanted their children to like. The children grew to like the foods their mothers introduced to them that way. Wouldn't it be so much easier on you and me if we had been trained to go the way of healthy food choices early in life? Maintaining good health will be easier for your kids if you help them make healthy choices while they are young.

Try resurrecting your appetite, and help your kids be healthy and wise by training your palate to like God-made foods. It won't take long. Isaiah 57:19 says God creates the fruit of our lips (and fruit is a good thing). Add these words to your training program as a kind of positive confession: "I am God's child, and I like God's foods. God's foods are good foods, so I like good foods." That is more of a faith confession for some of us than for others, but it's true. Repeating it can work wonders in resurrecting your appetite.

THE SIGNIFICANCE
OF SIGNATURES

On one of my recorded teaching series "You Are What You Ate," I talk about the doctrine of signatures, which is a fascinating study all by itself. Signatures are features in the appearance of natural foods that indicate what part of the body the foods benefit. In other words, God designed foods that resemble the part of the body they help.

Signatures are especially significant in regard to vegetables because the connections are so obvious. Cut a carrot in cross sections. What do you see? A little circle in the center of the carrot with striations going out from it in all directions. It looks like an orange eyeball, or at least an orange iris. Sure enough, carrots are loaded with vitamin A, which is good for your eyes. After all, have you ever seen a rabbit wearing glasses? See, it works!

Cut a tomato in cross sections. See how it is made up of inside chambers like the heart? Sure enough, tomatoes are heart-smart. The same with apples; doesn't an apple look almost heart-shaped and heart-sized? Apples are heart-smart too, along with strawberries, which are also heart-shaped. Grapes look a lot like red blood cells. Sure enough, they are loaded with antioxidants.

The long, hollow tubes running the length of celery stalks resemble the veins and arteries in our circulatory system. Guess what celery is good for? Right, it keeps blood circulation flowing. Do you know anyone with high blood pressure? Tell them to eat celery. The medicinal effects of eating three celery sticks a day may surpass any high blood pressure medication on the market!

The doctrine of signatures applies to other healthy foods. Walnuts and pecans with their fissured halves look kind of like your brain. You guessed it—nuts contain essential fatty acids that are healthy for the brain. At our house we eat nuts every day for brain power.

Kidney beans are kidney-shaped, of course, and they add fiber to your diet and help with waste elimination. A quarter cup a day of almost any kind of beans could lower your cholesterol by 19 percent. Add three raw carrots a day to that (also tube-shaped, like your blood vessels), and bad cholesterol is likely to decline another 11 percent, for an amazing 30 percent reduction in bad cholesterol levels—just from eating two vegetables!

WHAT'S THE BIG IDEA?

Fruits and veggies are amazingly healthy, yet 20 percent of Americans eat no vegetables and 40 percent eat no fruits. I'm not even talking fresh produce here, but *none* of any kind. Of the veggies Americans do consume, 25 percent are french fries—if you can even call those veggies. I sure can't, and that's not even taking into account the sodium and fat from the vats of grease used to fry them.

What are we Americans largely eating instead of fruits and vegetables? Fat- and chemical-laden fast foods with no nutritional value. Not surprisingly, these nutritionally void creations make us fat faster and sick more often. Hooked on convenience, even at home far too many Americans reach for premade dinners that originated in a factory-filled box, can, or freezer bag. These dinners have had the vitamins, minerals, and other healthy ingredients processed out and preservatives, false flavorings, and fake texturizers processed in. What is the big idea behind these phony ingredients? Profits, not health. Why do we keep on eating this way? Because millions of TV advertisements tell us to, and we think these man-made "foods" taste good and save us time.

I believe the irresponsible use of popular prepared foods has had a profoundly negative impact on America's physical health. I could fill more than one book with fire-and-brimstone preaching about the sad state of America's eating habits. Besides seasonal affective disorder, it is amazingly appropriate that the acronym SAD can also mean the standard American diet!

However, I prefer the positive approach. What's my philosophy? My big idea and calling is to markedly enhance the physical condition of fellow believers (and anyone else in our society who will listen) through creative teaching about biblical health. My goal is to make a difference not a buck. And a leading way to make a difference in your health and the health of your family is to bring on the fruits and vegetables.

BE CREATIVE!

While it may seem like the impossible dream in our convenience-oriented, fatty-food-advertising-saturated world, you *can* train yourself and your kids to crave fresh fruits and veggies in place of sweet and salty junk foods with no nutritive value. Use a little creativity. Cut up some of the fruits and vegetables I have mentioned, and show your kids the significance of their signatures. Tell them they are making their brains, eyes, and hearts strong and healthy when they eat foods designed to look like those parts of their bodies. Challenge them to examine natural foods and see if they can figure out what anatomical systems or organs they might benefit. Believe me, your kids will be fascinated and want to try new fruits and veggies.

Another method is to arrange cut-up fruit and veggie pieces attractively on a tray (eye appeal is buy appeal) and add a dish of healthy dip, such as vanilla yogurt for fruit or hummus (blended chickpeas) for vegetables. When you pop in a video, let the kids eat cherry tomatoes, celery, carrot sticks, and cucumbers while they watch. Make it your goal to eat a minimum of two to three servings of fruit and five to seven servings of vegetables daily. Remember, a suggested serving size is not that big, so this many servings is likely less than you may envision.

As I said, Susan and I try to compose 50 percent of our family's diet from these power-packed foods. Put a little time and ingenuity into resurrecting your family's appetite to a new healthy diet based on fruits and vegetables. The time and effort is well spent. It will yield healthy results a hundredfold!

SIMPLE YET PROFOUND: RESURRECT YOUR APPETITE

If you have been stuck in a high-fat, high-sugar eating routine, switching to lots of fruits and vegetables may sound like a thankless, impossible task. Yet sometimes eating healthy comes down to acquiring a taste for what is good for you. I promise this next statement is true, even though it sounds unbelievable: your body *will* crave God-made foods that are good for you if you give them the chance. It is just a matter of resurrecting your appetite.

Common sense says that since God wants us to live an abundant, joyful life, and since He created certain foods to fuel our bodies, we should also be *designed* to enjoy those foods, right? We are! However, some of us have forgotten how to enjoy God-made foods because we are overwhelmed with cravings for the wrong foods. Our bodies *will* crave whatever we feed them. We just need to feed our bodies the right things!

We all experience food cravings. How can we resurrect our appetites so our bodies crave God-made foods instead of man-made? Start with a little step of faith. One time we were invited to present our health seminar at a church in New York. After the Sunday morning service, Susan and I went to lunch with the pastor and his wife. The pastor decided then and there to take a small step toward resurrecting his appetite. We ate a buffet-style meal. Susan loaded her plate with carrots, cucumbers, and fruits—all healthy, God-made foods. The pastor looked at Susan's plate and then at his own, piled high with not-so-healthy choices. Then he looked back at Susan's plate again. I could see the wheels of his mind turning as he considered the material he had heard us present that morning.

"Susan, can I see your plate a second?" he finally asked my wife.

"Sure," Susan responded, gracious but puzzled.

He moved his own plate to the side, grabbed Susan's plate, and placed it in front of himself.

"How does that look?" he asked his wife. "Do you think I could get used to that?"

His wife laughed and shook her head a little at the unusual sight. At least he was experimenting to see how a plate of God-made food looked in place of his usual fare. Susan made him try a cucumber before he handed her plate back.

You may dislike certain foods right now—particularly certain fruits and vegetables—but if you know they're good for you and you start to eat them, you will soon find yourself craving them. Amazingly, God designed you that way. He is the ultimate Engineer. His work in designing your body and your appetite will pass the test. Try it!

At another church where we presented our seminar, the pastor told us his story about going on a short-term mission trip. A friend advised him to eat plenty of yogurt before leaving because yogurt is filled with *Lactobacillus acidophilus*, or "friendly" bacteria that promote intestinal health. His buddy said he was likely to encounter some unfriendly bacteria where he was headed, so he had to prepare ahead of time by giving his body the tools it needed to ward off illness.

"I never liked yogurt before the mission trip," the pastor told me. "I hated it so much that I had to plug my nose to eat it. Now I eat yogurt all the time, and I like it. I can't believe it!"

Granted, yogurt is not a fruit or vegetable such as I have been talking about. But natural yogurt is wonderful food, and this story illustrates my point—you *can* resurrect your healthy appetite. Get started today in retraining yourself by putting some healthy options into your diet.

CHAPTER 8

KEY 8:
BREAD FROM HEAVEN

I SUSPECT MANY MODERN-DAY Christians don't appreciate what strange birds God's prophets were, or what kind of faith it took to obey His directions. Take Isaiah, who walked around naked and barefoot for three years as a sign against Egypt and Ethiopia (if you don't believe me, read Isaiah 20:2-6). He told Elijah to walk before the most powerful ruler in Israel and proclaim that it wouldn't rain for the next three years because of the land's wickedness. Sound easy? Try making that kind of proclamation to the mayor of your city, let alone the president of the country. Another time God commanded Ezekiel to strikingly illustrate the siege of Jerusalem. He gave Ezekiel specific instructions about how to do this, telling him to lie on his left side for 390 days.

OK, head down to the city square for the next thirteen months and try doing this. Remember, you will have to survive for that long on the rations of bread and water prescribed for Ezekiel. In addition, you will need to cook your bread using the fuel God told him to use: human excrement. After the first day or two you would probably get arrested, if not for loitering, then for disturbing the peace and violating health codes. Of course, many people wouldn't be that concerned about the law. They would be busy asking, "What, no cheeseburgers? No steak? No baked potatoes? At least a slice of pizza? For heaven's sake, not even some carrots, broccoli, and an apple or two?"

Being a prophet was tough business. However, don't get too side-tracked over the limited menu God spelled out. Focus more on the fact that to insure His servant's survival, He gave him a recipe for the kind of bread that would sustain his life: "Take wheat, barley, beans, lentils, millet, and spelt, and put them into one vessel and make bread of them," God instructed. "According to the number of the days that you shall lie upon your side, 390 days you shall eat of it" (Ezek. 4:9, AMP).

Ezekiel bread. Sounds hearty, doesn't it? You can survive on bread like that. Have you ever tasted it? Before going further, let me say that I'm not being paid to promote Ezekiel 4:9 (which besides bread comes in a variety of buns, cereals, muffins, tortillas, and other products). I just happen to believe that it is simply the best whole-grain bread ever produced—not surprising, since the recipe comes straight out of the Bible. Ezekiel bread's popularity is on the rise and available in numerous stores and bakeries. I will caution you that it costs a lot more than the average loaf of white bread. Stack it up against its cheaper cousin, though. You will find twice the protein, nearly six times the fiber, no sugar (most commercial white bread has just over a gram), and no sodium, next to 170 milligrams in a slice of white bread. Although it has a few more calories, it has three times the potassium and 40 percent less fat.

I will grant you that the prophet Ezekiel may have tired of the taste after eating this bread day after day after day. Still, he lived on it for *390 days* (along with water), so it really is food capable of sustaining life. And it's good. Generally speaking, whole grains are more than good: they are the undisputed kings of high-fiber foods.

One of the ingredients in Ezekiel bread is millet, which Susan loves. Millet alone can sustain life. If all you had was millet and water, you would be all right. Not familiar with millet? Grab a handful of birdseed from your garage and take a look. Millet is the little, round grain contained in birdseed. Why throw all the good stuff to the birds? We ought to be eating millet too. In our house we do eat a form of birdseed every day by buying breads, cereals, and pastas with millet in their list of ingredients.

About now you may be thinking, "Great, this doctor wants us to relax, breathe deeply, and eat birdseed." I promise you that it beats embracing the alternative of living a stressed-out lifestyle, lacking fresh air and sunshine, and eating nonnutritious foods that sap your strength instead of supplying it. Even if it means eating birdseed now and again, "doing the dos" in my Ten Keys That Cure will bless and strengthen you!

This chapter reviews the first of the final three of my ten keys: whole grains. The others are pure water (which also sustained Ezekiel) and what the Bible calls "clean" meats. God once told another prophet Elijah to go into hiding for protection, and God commanded ravens to feed him. Elijah "went and stayed by the Brook Cherith, which flows into the Jordan. The ravens brought him bread and meat in the morning, and bread and meat in the evening; and he drank from the brook" (1 Kings 17:5–6). This is another example of a prophet living on bread and water, this time with a little meat thrown in (well, flown in). God knew these foods would sustain His prophets. They will sustain us as well.

WHOLE GRAINS

While you can consume grains in many forms, when most of us think of grains, we think of bread. When most of us think of bread, the first loaf that comes to mind is feathery-soft white bread. Did you know white bread is the most frequently purchased item in grocery stores? That is because it's a staple of SAD—the standard American diet—(and that *is* sad). White bread is simply not a staple at our house, and it shouldn't be at yours either. Why buy SAD white bread when you can buy bread made with the happy whole grains God created to nourish you?

You may wonder, "Why whole-grain bread? It's heavier and more expensive. I can get white bread for less than a dollar a loaf at the day-old bread store!" That line of thinking brings me to the next verse of "Dr. Don's Be Healthy Song."

> Please don't eat that white bread,
> The good nutrition's gone.
> Whole-wheat, rye, and good brown bread
> Will make you big and strong.

While it is true that whole-grain breads tend to be a little heavier in texture, that is a good thing. Once you taste their flavor and realize how satisfying they are, you will never go back to the cheap imitation! Again, it's a matter of training your palate to appreciate God-made foods, which make you feel healthier.

The only thing white bread does for you is leave a mass of gluey glop in your stomach. Try this sometime—put two pieces of soft, white bread in a bowl and add a little water. Then stir it up. What does it remind you of? That's right: glue. White bread is made from bleached or enriched flour, which means all the nutrition has been sucked out of the flour. Manufacturers then add sugar and loads of preservatives to keep that appealing but unhealthy loaf "fresh" on store shelves.

What's worse, *enriched* is a huge misnomer. Enriched flour has had most of the natural vitamins and minerals removed from it to give the bread a finer texture and longer shelf life. Your body absorbs it as a starch instead of a wheat or a grain, which it can use effectively for energy. Although it is enriched with B vitamins and iron, it lacks the vitamin E, natural fiber, and healthy trace minerals that are found in whole wheat flour. Goods made with this processed flour contain more empty calories than products made with whole wheat.

If this isn't enough to persuade you that white bread isn't very healthy, did you know that even rats—who will eat anything—cannot survive on it? When scientists tried feeding laboratory rats exclusively on white bread, guess what happened? They proved there's truth in the old saying, "The whiter the bread, the sooner you're dead." The rats died. Quickly. There was literally nothing left in white bread to keep them alive. One reason manufacturers enrich flour is to prevent bugs from eating it. Ironically, like rats, the bugs will die if they try to make dinner from it.

With bread and other baked products, beware of any ingredients that include the words *bleached, enriched,* or *fortified.* Those words mean all the good, healthy fibers such as grain husks have been removed from these processed products and fed to farm animals. While these animals do all right, when we eat the leftovers in the form of white bread, we suffer ill health. Did you know that God indicated that overprocessing grain damages it? "Grain for bread is crushed. Indeed, he [the farmer] does not continue to thresh it forever. Because the wheel of his cart and his horses eventually damage it, he does not thresh it any longer" (Isa. 28:28, NAS). In other words, process grain too much, and the good nutrition vanishes!

Instead of white bread at the grocery store, grab a 100 percent whole-grain bread, whether Ezekiel or some other kind. Here is a good rule of thumb when buying bread. Any loaf that you can easily crush should be left at the store. However, that doesn't mean you should visit the bread aisle and leave a trail of crumpled bread bags in your wake (the store manager may kick you out in a hurry). Still, give that loaf you're about to put into your cart a gentle squeeze. If you can't feel some solid texture between your fingertips, you will know there is nothing in there to nourish and sustain you. It isn't much more than air, sugar, and preservatives—in essence, a dessert. And not a very good one.

Whole grains are powerful health promoters. Ezekiel bread is a sprouted grain bread that even has some beans in it. As a result, it is high in fiber, which is great for your intestinal tract. That's important. As I said earlier, the road to health is paved with good intestines. I also discussed earlier how your colon must function well for you to stay healthy, and Ezekiel and other healthy whole-wheat breads will help.

You can incorporate whole grains into your diet in many appetizing ways. Try wheat, barley, rye, millet, or oats for starters. When Susan cooks up oatmeal for breakfast and tops it with blueberries, a touch of real maple syrup, and a dash of cinnamon, she says the taste reminds her of blueberry pie. At lunchtime we might have a turkey sandwich on whole-grain bread, and for dinner a bowl of barley soup hits the spot. Whole grains are wholly good for your health!

SIMPLE YET PROFOUND: READ THE LABEL

Another rule of thumb is to read the ingredients on the labels of bread and any other food. If you can't understand the label, or if it lists man-made ingredients instead of God-made ones, you are better off without it. Food ingredients are always listed in the order of amount; the most prominent one is at the top of the list, then the next, and so on. If bleached or enriched flour is ingredient number one and sugar is number two, leave that loaf like a bad habit. If you cannot decipher some of the ingredients, consider it a *warning* label, not a food label. Stop and drop. Forget that loaf and roll your cart over to one with a label you can understand.

This is why I follow the rule that if I can't understand an ingredient on a food label, I don't put it into my body! Avoiding preservatives is a leading way to preserve your life and improve your health. Consider the real-life example of a sign on a vending machine at a zoo. It read, "*PLEASE* do not feed vending-machine food to the animals—they might get sick and die!" Think about that next time your kids are standing in line at a vending machine full of overprocessed, overpreserved foods. We know better than to feed such foods to animals. Why in heaven's name would we want to stuff our kids, or ourselves, with them?

CHAPTER 9

KEY 9:
WHITE IF YOU EAT MEAT

IT IS TRUE that the first chapter of Genesis designates fruits, vegetables, and whole grains as human beings' source of food, just as it is true that God did not originally design us to be meat eaters. Our intestinal tracts most closely resemble that of herbivorous creatures, who have longer intestines with a low acid content. On the other hand, carnivores have shorter intestinal tracts and ten times the acid content. Still, this doesn't mean that the Bible insists that we must eat an exclusively vegetarian diet. Earlier I mentioned how God commanded ravens to sustain Elijah during a rough period with bread *and* meat.

Consider too what God told Noah and his sons in the ninth chapter of Genesis. After the flood He said, "All the animals of the earth, all the birds of the sky, all the small animals that scurry along the ground, and all the fish in the sea will look on you with fear and terror. I have placed them in your power. I have given them to you for food, just as I have given you grain and vegetables" (Gen. 9:2–3, NLT). After Noah and his family disembarked from the ark, God added meat to humankind's diet. He may have made this addition for a number of reasons. Presumably the flood would have destroyed all edible vegetation. It would have taken too much time for Noah and his family to plant and harvest crops. Perhaps they were in need of another source of nutrition. Whatever God's reasons, He told them they could eat meat; this practice has continued ever since.

The New Testament also mentions the permissibility of eating meat, when Paul warned Timothy to watch out for those who command others "to abstain from meats, which God hath created to be received with thanksgiving....For every creature of God is good, and nothing to be refused, if it be received with thanksgiving: For it is sanctified by the word of God and prayer" (1 Tim. 4:3–5, KJV).

This passage assures us that we can eat anything with prayer and thanksgiving. It is right and good to pray over our food—especially some of the stuff included in the standard American diet. Considering the plethora of fat, sugar, and sodium added to so many processed foods, we better be praying over those food choices! I confess Mark 16:18 over my rare cups of coffee: "If they [believers] drink any deadly thing, it shall not hurt them" (KJV).

DIETARY LAWS

In the Book of Leviticus God distinguished what meat choices were clean or unclean, warning the Israelites to avoid the latter. Even though today we are "not under law but under grace" (Rom. 6:14), those Levitical laws still pose important guidelines for healthy eating. Many Old Testament laws are still applicable today. Although we don't *have to* do them, we *get to* do them. We should do our best to follow them because our Creator's wisdom goes far beyond our own.

Scientific research continues to prove the validity of many Old Testament laws dealing with health and nutrition. One amazing example is God's instruction to separate people who carried an infection. No one in Old Testament times knew about viruses and bacteria, yet God provided His people with laws that would prevent the spread of infections. Epidemics raged through Egypt and other ancient cultures. Yet when the Israelites followed God's health instructions, they suffered none of those diseases.

The rest of us didn't catch on to the validity of some of the Old Testament's hygienic teachings until almost two hundred years ago, when Dr. Ignaz Semmelweis first suspected that medical students who didn't wash their hands were passing horrible infections from bodies in the autopsy room to women in maternity wards. In a Vienna hospital Semmelweis sternly ordered medical staff to wash their hands in a chlorinated solution before examining women in labor. Immediately the mortality rate of mothers under his care dropped drastically.

Despite this astonishing result, traditionalists ridiculed Semmelweis for his beliefs. In fact, they maligned him so severely that he eventually left his position and committed suicide. Time and research have since proven the wisdom of his observations and efficacy of his methods. Now that we can see these deadly germs through a microscope, we know why caution around infectious people makes good sense. Semmelweis was right all along, just as the Bible instructed before he came on the scene.

The same holds true with Old Testament laws regarding clean and unclean meats. God protected His people's health long before anyone understood the physiological reasons behind His rules. Even today it makes good health sense for many reasons to choose meats from the "clean" lists in the Old Testament and avoid unclean meats.

Clean animals are those that chew the cud and have split hooves, such as sheep, oxen, deer, and the like. Unclean animals are the scavenger sorts; for example, fish without fins and scales, certain birds, and pigs. The eleventh chapter of Leviticus reviews clean and unclean meats. Because of the instruction in verses 7–8, Jewish people have long been known to avoid pork. I'm with them on that! Why? Because pigs eat anything and everything in sight, meaning they accumulate astronomic levels of toxins in their tissues. Pork meat actually rots from the inside out, not the outside in. That alone ought to tell us pork is definitely not "the other white meat"!

As for sea creatures, Leviticus 11:9 says that the healthiest to consume are those with fins and scales. Why are they clean? Fins and scales mean they are moving through the water, whereas creatures without fins and scales are probably bottom dwellers such as lobsters (called the "cockroaches of the sea") and crabs. These bottom feeders filter the water, consume refuse, and accumulate toxins in their tissues in the same way that pigs consume trash on land.

WHERE'S THE BEEF?

What about beef? An occasional meal of red meat is all right. Indeed, lean, hormone-free beef can be healthier than cage-raised chicken with the skin left on. Still, beef should not be a part of every main meal. If you were brought up on beef, as many of us were, it is wise to limit beef consumption to once a week. Once every two weeks is even better. Once you get used to that restriction, cut back to once a month. That may seem extreme in our beef-crazed culture, but when you're eating a healthy, tasty variety of other meats, you won't be asking, "Where's the beef?" nearly as often as you think.

Limiting your overall consumption of meat and dairy products is a good idea anyway. Modern factory farms typically confine cattle in tight spaces, increase their fat content with corn and other grains, and then pump them full of growth hormones and antibiotics to ward off diseases that stem from this unhealthy diet and environment. Sixty percent of all the antibiotics used in the United States are given to animals, which means when you consume a lot of meat and dairy products, you are ingesting unhealthy side effects of the food industry's profit-driven efficiencies.

The danger of consuming too many antibiotics is that you kill the good bacteria as well as the bad bacteria in your body systems. You desperately need that good bacteria at work inside you. You can replenish it by eating yogurt, apples, cabbage, figs, pineapples, and prunes.

You may have heard of some people developing immunity to many antibiotics, which means their doctors have a hard time finding something to prescribe for them when they're ill. The cause isn't necessarily all the antibiotics they have directly taken in the past; it's all the antibiotics they ingest indirectly by eating animal products.

This doesn't mean you can never go to a wonderful seafood buffet, order a juicy beefsteak, or eat a fast-food cheeseburger. However, it does mean that such choices should not characterize your daily diet. Remember, God said to worship Him in spirit and in truth, not at the drive-up window booth!

Proverbs 23:20 (KJV) warns, "Be not among winebibbers; among riotous eaters of flesh." If you are not among them, you won't be one of them! Who are these "riotous eaters of flesh"? They are gluttons when it comes to eating meat. Sadly, most Americans fall into that category. Proverbs goes on to say, "The drunkard and the glutton will come to poverty, and drowsiness will clothe a man with rags" (v. 21). Ever feel drowsy after a huge meal—or, if you've been down that road—drinking too much alcohol? Both practices literally put you in a stupor.

In the Bible, eating meat typically occurred at celebrations. Back then people did not eat meat every day—and certainly not three times a day, as many Americans do. People saved meat for special occasions. When the prodigal son returned home, his father told his servants to "kill the calf we have been fattening. We must celebrate with a feast" (Luke 15:23, NLT). In the past you may have missed the significance of this verse. Namely, the fatted calf was a treat, not an everyday meal! It is best to moderate your meat consumption and learn the facts about the meats you eat.

In place of red beef, when it comes to meat, look for the white—but not pork. At our house we like fish, chicken, and turkey, primarily because they are lower in fat. Excess fat is where the toxins accumulate. For that reason, by the way, meat preparation is nearly as important as meat choice. If you leave on the skin, where most of the fat is, and fry the meat, you greatly increase the fat content. Lean, skinless cuts are the way to go!

I particularly like fish. Jesus set a good example for us in John 21:9-13 when He cooked the disciples fish for breakfast. Like Him, we should eat the healthiest meat most often. Jesus served His disciples the best of everything spiritually and physically. Not only is fish packed with nutrition, but it also contains good fats and oils that lubricate your joints while boosting your immune system and brain function.

One additional word about meat: it is a good idea to avoid red meat in particular because of its fat content. When God spelled out various dietary and sacrificial laws in Leviticus, He told them "all the fat is the Lord's" (Lev. 3:16), and then followed with these words: "This shall be a perpetual statute throughout your generations in all your dwellings: you shall eat neither fat nor blood" (v. 17). Perpetual means forever—in every generation and every home, none of God's people were ever to eat fat or blood. God gave that strict, perpetual command not because He was a killjoy, but because He wanted to protect His people's health. If you refrain from fat and blood, it will protect your health too!

ARE EGGS "EGG-CEPTABLE"?

Whenever I lead seminars and review guidelines for protein-rich foods such as meat, the discussion invariably comes around to eggs. The scare over the cholesterol in eggs has made them into the topic of fear and avoidance in "healthy" diets. However, no one should avoid eggs. After all, the Bible mentions them in such passages as Luke 11:11–13: "If a son asks for bread from any father among you, will he give him a stone? Or if he asks for a fish, will he give him a serpent instead of a fish? Or if he asks for an egg, will he offer him a scorpion? If you then, being evil, know how to give good gifts to your children, how much more will your heavenly Father give the Holy Spirit to those who ask Him!"

This Scripture passage suggests to me that bread, fish, and eggs are *good* gifts (at least as opposed to stones, serpents, and scorpions). Just as fish is healthy, so are eggs. Never mind the cholesterol—God put nutrients like lecithin into eggs to emulsify, or help your body metabolize, that cholesterol. Besides, eggs are loaded with B vitamins and contain choline, which converts to acetylcholine in your body. That is the memory transmitter in your brain. Earlier I mentioned the adage "an apple a day keeps the doctor away" and that two per day would keep him away twice as long. To that I would add that an egg a day helps your brain work the right way.

Eggs are a wonderful, God-made food. Man cannot duplicate the egg. Don't fall for those "egg substitutes" poured out of a carton. They aren't much more than egg whites with artificial color added (and that is definitely not good for you). If you want to eat only egg whites, which are complete proteins by themselves, then separate the yolks and throw them away. That is the inexpensive way to make egg substitutes—but why would you? I always eat the yolk and white of an egg. Yolks are loaded with nutrition because God designed them that way. It is always best to eat God-made foods the way He made them, without processing them to death or taking out all the nutrients.

These divine principles of nutrition from both the Old and New Testaments still work in favor of your health. So try some Ezekiel bread and other whole-grain foods, eat an egg every day, consider fats an offering to God, and skip the unclean meats while choosing white instead. Like the Israelites, you will reap the benefits of biblical good health when you apply biblical nutritional principles to food choices.

SIMPLE YET PROFOUND: GET HOOKED ON FISH

If you are not a fish-eater, introducing fish into your daily diet can seem like quite a chore. My first advice is to choose fresh first, frozen second, and canned sparingly. The Old Testament dietary laws have good advice about which seafood to eat. The good fish are those that swim and have scales and fins, such as salmon, tilapia, halibut, perch, orange roughy, and tuna. These are clean fish that move through the water.

Meanwhile, such "delicacies" as crab, lobster, and shrimp are bottom-feeding scavengers. While they served a positive purpose for the oceans in acting as their natural filters, the Old Testament prohibited God's people from eating them! I think it is wise to pay attention to this dietary guideline.

Two ways my family enjoys fish are when I broil it on tinfoil in the oven or sauté it in a little olive oil on top of the stove. Squeezing a little lemon juice over it or topping it with tomatoes during cooking can allay some of the fishy flavor.

Here is a recipe for oven-fried fish that will tickle your tastebuds. Change it as you desire with your favorite seasonings, herbs, and spices.

Easy Oven-Fried Fish

2 lbs. fish fillets
1 Tbsp. lemon juice
¼ cup fat-free milk
2 Tbsp. hot pepper sauce
1 tsp. fresh minced garlic
¼ Tbsp. each of salt, pepper, and onion powder
½ cup whole-wheat bread crumbs (make them from the
  crust ends)
1 Tbsp. olive oil for greasing baking dish
1 fresh lemon, cut into wedges

Preheat oven to 475°. Wipe fillets with lemon juice and pat dry. Combine milk, hot pepper sauce, and garlic. Combine pepper, salt, and onion powder with bread crumbs and place on a plate. Let fillets sit in milk briefly. Remove and coat fillets on both sides with seasoned crumbs. Let stand briefly until coating sticks to each side of fish. Arrange on lightly oiled shallow baking dish. Bake 20 minutes on middle rack without turning. Cut into 6 pieces. Serve with fresh lemon.

CHAPTER 10

KEY 10:
WATER OF LIFE

Y OU COULD SAY that health starts with a five-letter word: W-A-T-E-R. Your body is mostly made of water—between 65 and 70 percent. Your brain is more than 80 percent water, and your blood is more than 90 percent water. Since "the life of the flesh is in the blood" (Lev. 17:11), you need water, water, and more water to be healthy.

Through breathing, urination, and sweating, you lose approximately 64 ounces of water a day. This means you need to drink eight 8-ounce glasses of water just to break even and replenish yourself. Few people break even—most people drink much less. I cannot overestimate the number of people who walk around chronically dehydrated!

Do you often feel fatigued, irritable, depressed, confused, or beset by intense food cravings? You could simply be dehydrated. You can do a couple easy self-tests to check. First, lightly pinch the skin on the back of your hand together and pull upward. If your skin doesn't immediately recede back into place when you let go, but stays raised for a few seconds, you need more water. Second, check the color of your urine. It should be light, not dark or yellow. If your urine is colored, you need to drink more water.

Dehydration creates a multitude of physical problems. It gives illness and disease a chance to take hold in your body. Many illnesses are exacerbated by, or even result from, chronic dehydration. Often, when the doctor diagnoses an illness, you're not so much *sick* as you are *thirsty*. The medical community often ends up treating the effects of pitifully low water intake with medication. However, many medications can poison your body and generate undesirable side effects, so you want to avoid them as much as possible. In large part, you can accomplish that by drinking the water your body so desperately needs. A well-hydrated body is a healthy body.

If you significantly increase water intake, your sensitivity to your body's need for water will also multiply. The more water you give your body, the more you will know when you need it. That is a good way to start a healthy cycle.

As a doctor, if I were forced to pick only two ways to improve health, I would choose increasing water and fiber intake. It is hard to believe what a difference those two steps can make. Remember, half the health equation is detoxification (the other half is balancing the immune system). Water is the ultimate detoxifier. If you aren't getting enough, an increase of only five glasses a day may cut the risk of colon cancer by 45 percent, bladder cancer by 50 percent, and breast cancer by 79 percent. Cancer can only develop in an acidic environment. Guess what dehydration does? Causes your body to be acidic. Many people live on the cusp of acidity—a real risk to health—but the more water you drink, the more balanced your pH levels.

Water also acts as a powerful cleanser to remove plaque from artery walls. It is instrumental in stabilizing blood pressure. In addition, water lubricates the joints to prevent arthritis and diminishes headaches. Dehydration can cause all kinds of painful symptoms;

water can decrease them all—or even make them disappear. Here is another health equation:

More water = less disease

I believe 50 percent of our nation's health problems would disappear if we drank enough water. That's why "Dr. Don's Be Healthy Song" water verse goes:

Water cleans your body
Outside and within.
Eight glasses a day is the natural way
For cleansing to begin.

Notice that eight glasses *begins* the cleansing. You need more water than that, but I originally composed this song for children, who need a little less.

In chapter 8 I talked about the vast health benefits of the bread recipe God gave to the prophet Ezekiel. God also commanded him to drink water: "You shall also drink water by measure, one-sixth of a hin; from time to time you shall drink" (Ezek. 4:11)—a *hin* being about a gallon. Then there was Elijah, to whom the ravens brought meat. God commanded Elijah to "hide by the Brook Cherith, which flows into the Jordan. And it will be that you shall drink from the brook" (1 Kings 17:3-4). If God commanded His prophets to drink water from time to time throughout the day, it is probably a good idea for you and me too!

HOW MUCH WATER
DO YOU NEED?

Many people do not relish drinking water. If you are one of them, take heart. Your appreciation for this liquid nourishment will increase if you will just start drinking it. To enhance its taste, try adding a slice of lemon or lime, as well as cooling your water in summer or warming it in winter. However, skip sugary powdered drink mixes, hot chocolate, and coffee. None of these have the same health benefits of water—quite the opposite. I will explain why shortly.

First, here is a simple way to figure out how much water you need daily. Divide your weight in pounds by two and drink that many ounces of water. If you weigh 150 pounds, divide by two to get your recommended intake of 75 ounces a day—about ten 8-ounce cups. This will help at least replenish what you are losing. Once you are used to that amount, drink some more!

I know some of you are thinking, "Wow, that's a lot of water—I'll be drowning in it!" It isn't that hard to drink all you need if you try these suggestions: Start with a glass or two as soon as you wake up. You will soon get used to it and even miss it if you skip this wake-up beverage. Drink a glass or two right before meals too. This helps fill your stomach, enabling you to eat moderately and maintain your ideal weight. Take water along in the car and drink it at stoplights. Keep water on your desk at work. The more it is readily available, the more you will drink. Before you know it, it will become a healthy habit. If you have suffered from dehydration, you will feel ten times better than you do right now.

WHAT KIND OF WATER?

People often ask, "What *kind* of water should I drink?" You may think that water is water. Not true. There is tap water, bottled water, flavored water, reverse-osmosis water, and purified water. The list goes on and on. To the oft-asked question—"Should I drink tap water?"—the answer is a resounding, "No!" At least not if you have another source. If you don't, then undoubtedly the health benefits of drinking tap water (even with all the chemicals in it) outweigh the detriments of not drinking enough water. Any water is far better than no water.

However, the way tap water is processed in most municipalities leaves it full of chemicals, particularly chlorine and fluoride. Have you ever looked at your bathwater and noticed it was blue? Or taken a drink from your tap and thought, "This tastes like the swimming pool water I swallowed by accident?" Take the hint—water that looks, smells, and tastes bad *is* bad. Besides, drinking water should make you want more, not make you grimace at every swallow.

One alternative is bottled water, which is available almost everywhere. You are better off choosing water in a plastic bottle than soda pop (whether in a bottle or a can) any day. However, getting attached to those plastic containers isn't wise, especially if you get into the habit of repeatedly refilling the bottles.

While you may be making a well-intentioned effort to increase your water intake, reusing bottles will increase ingestion of harmful chemicals that leach into water from plastic. Reusing bottles accelerates the leaching process, since more chemicals leach into a beverage from a reused plastic bottle than a new one. Drink bottled water when it is the best choice available, but save yourself a glass bottle of some sort if you like refills.

Although flavored waters are increasing in popularity—many labels list water, 100 percent natural fruit flavors, and zero calories—watch out for their hazards. Just like diet drinks, most also contain artificial sweeteners, which will poison you. (I will talk more about soft drinks shortly.) Some flavored waters are also carbonated. I'm not a big fan of carbonation because it acidifies your body, setting you up for all kinds of disease. If you crave strawberry-flavored water, instead of buying flavored water, slice up a *real* strawberry and put it in a glass of water. Cucumber water is delicious and refreshing too. Almost any restaurant will serve you a slice of lemon or lime in your water if you request it. Make your own flavored waters with natural ingredients.

Overall, purified water is the best. We personally like reverse-osmosis filtration or carbon filtration. Sometimes we use steam-distilled water. A reverse-osmosis water system is an excellent investment in your health. Reverse osmosis is a safe, effective way to remove the most common toxins found in water.

The important thing, though, is to use some type of filtration system. If all you can afford is a $20, sit-on-the-counter type water filter from the grocery store, buy one today. It will filter out 98 or 99 percent of the impurities in tap water and vastly improve the taste. One way or another, supply yourself and your family with a source of fresh, purified water.

DO OTHER DRINKS COUNT?

What about all those other drinks in your fridge or pantry? Can they count as part of your water intake? Absolutely not. You want to avoid most other drinks that are part of the standard American diet. Nothing can take the place of water. Most other drinks on the market do you far more harm than good. If you knew what happens inside your body when you drink some of them, you would demand the containers be labeled with a skull and crossbones!

Take coffee, for example. How many coffee addicts do you know? It is one thing to get up and start the day with this favorite beverage (after you drink your water, of course). It is quite another to get up and get hit by a nagging headache because you haven't had your caffeine fix. As if this addiction weren't bad enough, drinking coffee also causes an excessive loss of vital calcium through urination and increases the risk of cadmium toxicity. Both caffeinated and decaffeinated coffee contain cadmium, which promotes cancerous cell changes. Natural alternatives to coffee are much safer. For an energy boost and focused thinking, try green tea, ginkgo biloba, and ginseng drinks.

As for soft drinks, there is nothing *soft* about them. They are *hard* on your body! The excess sugar and phosphates cause calcium loss, and the sugar turns to fat and depletes your body of B vitamins. Sugar (in soft drinks or anything else) also depresses your immune system by lowering white blood cell activity. Ever wonder why there is a higher incidence of colds and flu during the holiday season? Maybe low resistance to holiday treats and low resistance to illnesses are related.

Soft drinks also knock off your pH balance, acidify your body, and promote aging and free-radical damage. The pH level of colas ranges between 2.7 and 3.4. Normal is 7.0. Think about this: if you drop a tooth into a cup of cola, that tooth will completely dissolve in ten days! No wonder trucks carrying colas are required to put "Highly Corrosive!" signs on their tanks. Do you want that kind of acid working its way through your body? You need to drink more than thirty-two glasses of pure water to undo the nasty effects of one soft drink! Are you willing to fill up that can or bottle thirty-two times with water and drink it all to alleviate the impact of one cola?

Diet soft drinks are no better. In fact, they are worse. Artificial sweeteners in diet drinks and other foods are highly toxic. Any time those sweeteners get above eighty-six degrees—and your body temperature is normally twelve degrees hotter than that—they break down into three poisonous substances:

- One is methanol (methyl alcohol). Toxic levels of this substance cause blindness.

- Another is formic acid. This is what poisonous insects inject into you. Why do it to yourself?

- The third is cancer-causing formaldehyde.

These aren't substances you want roving around inside you. And forget losing any pounds—with consistent use, artificial sweeteners actually cause weight gain! Think it over. After three decades of active marketing of diet soft drinks, the average weight of people in our society has gone up, not down. Obviously we're not getting any smaller. However, we are suffering from obesity and diseases such as diabetes much more frequently.

Finally, what about alcohol? Did you know the Bible specifically warns thirty-eight times against alcohol abuse? It is a poison that directly damages the brain, liver, pancreas, and small intestine. The danger of killing brain cells is self-explanatory. A damaged liver is prey to hepatitis and cirrhosis. Pancreas damage ushers in diabetes. Small intestine problems lead to poor absorption of all nutrients, especially fat-soluble vitamins (A, D, E, and K), B vitamins, folic acid, and vitamin C. Many of these nutrients are meant to protect the body from free-radical damage that promotes aging and aging-related diseases such as heart disease, cancer, and arthritis. These nutrients can't protect you if your body can't absorb them.

Alcohol increases free-radical formation, which makes it a two-edged sword that points towards aging. Ever notice how alcohol abusers often look much older than their chronological age? Those who routinely consume alcohol suppress their immune systems and age themselves prematurely. In addition, just two or more drinks of alcoholic beverages a day increase a person's chances of developing tumor growths by an almost unbelievable 80 percent!

You may be wondering, "If alcohol is so bad for you, then why is it so widely known that drinking some red wine every day is supposed to be beneficial to your health?" There is a nutritional reason behind that finding that has nothing to do with the wine. When red wine is made by crushing grapes, the grape skins and seeds are left in during the process. People today are generally so nutrient-depleted that those who drink red wine actually benefit not from the wine itself, but the nutrients in the grape skins and seeds. You can gain the same exact benefit from red or purple grape juice. Don't fall for the "red wine is good for you" slogan as an excuse to consume alcohol. There is no good reason to risk your health by consuming alcohol.

I should note that my family and I enjoy other healthy beverages in addition to water. There is even one drink that counts toward recommended daily water consumption—green tea. You can drink four cups of green tea daily in place of four cups of water. I drink about six cups of green tea daily. It is loaded with health benefits. Manufacturers are now cashing in on that discovery. You can buy green tea soaps, shampoos, and even green tea ice cream—although I wouldn't recommend the latter daily! Nor would I recommend buying green tea in plastic bottles at the store. It is usually loaded with either sugar or artificial sweeteners and other unhealthy additives. Stick to the kind you can brew yourself.

At our house we also like herb teas and fresh vegetable or fruit juices, or sometimes bottled juices with no additives. Since our bodies are mostly water, though, we drink what we're mostly made of. As my song concludes, water makes your health complete!

YOU'RE FEELING BETTER ALREADY

We have covered a lot of ground in this book. We have explored all Ten Keys That Cure, found them in the pages of Scripture, and illustrated how to apply them in everyday life. You have learned how to four-six it (Phil. 4:6) and cast all your cares on the Lord so you can relax. You have rediscovered the importance of a good night's rest (early to bed, early to rise). You have grappled with that infamous "E" word, *exercise*, and seen how beneficial it is to incorporate a little walking into your lifestyle. You know that fresh air and sunshine are good for you; they brighten your day and your mental outlook.

From a nutritional standpoint, you now know that it is possible to resurrect your appetite for healthy, God-made foods. You can train your palate and your family's to enjoy fresh fruits and vegetables. You were designed to enjoy them! You can buy whole-grain Ezekiel bread at the grocery store and add in a little clean meat on the side. God said all these things are to be enjoyed with thanksgiving. You can drink, drink, drink water and learn to love it (while praying Mark 16:18—that no deadly drink will harm you—over some of your other beverage choices).

With all this simple, practical information at your fingertips, you may be feeling better already! I hope learning about my Ten Keys

That Cure has helped you. Even if you pick only one key at a time and apply it, your health will take a turn for the better. Every believer can enjoy biblical good health. You have learned how through the pages of God's Word. His marvelous health plan *will* work for you.

In the next chapter I will review some related health questions that always come up in my seminars and other presentations. Do you wonder about when to see a doctor? How about the necessity of vitamins and other supplements? What about cholesterol? And how can you check for yourself whether you are in good health? I will address these questions and other health issues. Your health is your choice. I hope to help you choose the good life!

SIMPLE YET PROFOUND: SING A LITTLE SONG

Before she retired, my mother taught school. She once had a classroom full of busy second-graders to whom she imparted her vast wisdom—when she wasn't drilling it into me at home. In her classroom I found my first platform for preaching about biblical health. Mom and my sister (also a second-grade teacher) invited me to come to school on career day and talk to the kids about the medical profession and good health. As I attempted to distill my medical and scriptural knowledge about health principles into a format second-graders could understand, the Lord helped simplify and clarify it in my mind. I ended up composing a little song that says it all.

That was more than twenty years ago, and it hasn't changed since. I'm still singing the same tune. Its chorus condenses my twenty-one years of school and twenty years of Bible study into a few simple lines. I wish I could share the melody with you through the pages of this book—once children hear the catchy tune, they rarely forget it.

Parents and grandparents who have bought our CD will attest that once children learn the song, adults can't get away with anything! I will share the chorus from "Dr. Don's Be Healthy Song" with you here:

> Learn to relax,
> Get to bed on time,
> And do your exercise.
> Breathe fresh air
> While the sun's out there,
> And eat like this little rhyme:
> Fruits and vegetables,
> Whole grains,
> White if you choose meat.
> Drink what you're mostly made of,
> Water makes your health complete.

The whole song contains more verses that elaborate on these Ten Keys That Cure. In a nutshell, though, if you "do the dos" in the chorus, you will enjoy great health and have all the energy you need to do the things God wants you to do.

CHAPTER 11

YOUR HEALTH IS YOUR CHOICE. CHOOSE LIFE!

THEY HAD JUST crossed the desert in a grueling, forty-year-long march. God had proven time and again that He would guide them through every obstacle and literally rain down food from heaven (whether manna or quail). Yet most of the Israelites doubted Him—to the point that of all adults over the age of twenty, only Joshua and Caleb survived. Near the end of their journey God delivers a lengthy message (Deut. 29–30) through Moses in which He tells them about the blessings of following His commands and then warns of the disastrous consequences of disobedience. He concludes, "Today I have given you the choice between life and death, between blessings and curses. Now I call on heaven and earth to witness the choice you make. Oh, that you would choose life, so that you and your descendants might live!" (Deut. 30:19, NLT).

God is still presenting His people, including you and me, with a multiple-choice test. We can choose A, life and blessings, or B, death and curses. Then God tells us the answer to the test: "Choose life!" It doesn't get any clearer than that. God gives us the choices and tells us what to choose to enjoy life.

Notice, however, that He doesn't force us to make the right choice.

He doesn't choose for us. He has given every person a free will, and He always respects that. Each of us must choose to live for God or for the devil, to eat for good health or for poor health, to go the easy way or go the way of disobedience, which is hard. (Ask anyone who has undergone painful surgery because of poor health habits.)

When we stick to God's healthy principles and eat God-made foods, we will reap the benefits God promises in His Word. Psalm 103:5 says it is the Lord "who satisfies your mouth with good things, so that your youth is renewed like the eagle's." Susan likes that thought—eat God-made "good things" and you will look and feel younger!

Exodus 23:25–26 promises, "So you shall serve the LORD your God, and He will bless your bread and water. And I will take sickness away from the midst of you. No one shall suffer miscarriage or be barren in your land; I will fulfill the number of your days." Our family uses the beginning of this verse as our prayer before every meal: "Thank You, Lord, for blessing our bread and water and taking sickness and disease from the midst of us. In Jesus's name, Amen." We love these promises.

What blessings God pours out on us when we serve Him and live His way in every area of life—including nutrition! He says He will bless the food we eat, take away sickness and disease, bless women in childbearing, and ensure that we live long lives. That is the best health care benefit package you can ever hope to find!

WHAT ABOUT SEEING A DOCTOR?

As we travel and teach, many people ask us, "What about seeing a doctor? Does 'doing the dos' and eating God-made foods mean I will never have to go to a physician?" Not necessarily. I am trained as a physician. The Bible calls Luke, who wrote the Gospel of Luke and the Book of Acts, "the beloved physician" (Col. 4:14). Believers see Jesus as the Great Physician who heals all our diseases—spirit, soul, and body. Jesus even talked about seeing doctors when He said, "It is not those who are healthy who need a physician, but those who are sick" (Luke 5:31, AMP).

Seeing a doctor regarding a health concern is not a sin. Nor does it necessarily show a lack of faith, but let me say this: the first doctor you should visit with any health issue is Dr. Jesus. You wouldn't believe the number of people who approach me about a health issue and when I ask, "Have you prayed about your situation?" stammer, "Uh, no, not really..." When I ask, "What verse are you standing on from God's Word about this issue?" most people can't give one. Approaching the Great Physician is often the last thing that comes to people's minds—the last resort, a desperate measure, so to speak—when it ought to be the first thing they do!

Three other doctors I recommend that you visit regularly are Dr. Diet, Dr. Quiet, and Dr. Merryman. Dr. Diet will tell you to eat the foods God created because "you are what you ate!" Your body is constantly changing—literally making itself new out of the foods you've eaten. For instance, every twenty-eight to forty-five days you have a brand-new skin. Your body "sheds" an astonishing forty pounds of dust over your lifetime in the form of skin particles (dander or dandruff) as your skin becomes new. Every six weeks you have a brand-new liver. It only takes three to five days for your stomach lining to be renewed (because of the high acid content, the cells are exchanged quickly). In a twelve-month period, 98 percent of your atoms and molecules are replaced, all manufactured from the foods you consume.

The question is: Do you want to turn out like a cream puff or become a factory-wrapped cupcake with no substance? Or do you want your body to be made of healthy, fresh, whole foods? You are what you ate!

Dr. Quiet will tell you to relax the way God modeled for us (and instructed us to follow) when He instituted a Sabbath day of rest. The Bible promises, "A calm and undisturbed mind and heart are the life and health of the body" (Prov. 14:30, AMP). That is one of my favorite health verses (of course, I have many favorites). It is healthy to stay calm and relaxed. Practice more than stress management—practice stress elimination by four-sixing it and casting all your cares on the One who cares for you. Get the rest and exercise you need to rejuvenate body, soul, and spirit, as Jesus did.

Dr. Merryman will quote Proverbs 17:22, "A merry heart does good, like medicine." Likewise, Proverbs 15:30 says, "A cheerful look brings joy to the heart, and good news gives health to the bones" (NIV). Put simply, happier people are healthier people. I'm sure that is a primary reason the apostle Paul advised, "Friends, I'd say you'll do best by filling your minds and meditating on things true, noble, reputable, authentic, compelling, gracious—the best, not the worst; the beautiful, not the ugly; things to praise, not things to curse" (Phil. 4:8, THE MESSAGE).

On the other hand, Proverbs 14:30 warns us that "envy, jealousy, and wrath are like rottenness of the bones" (AMP). Another version, the New Living, translates "rottenness" as "cancer." That is much too high a price to pay for harboring negative emotions. Get rid of any junk in your trunk such as negative emotions, anger, holding grudges toward others, and anxiety. Trust in God's promise of an abundant life, and as Paul emphasized by saying it again and again, "Rejoice in the Lord always. Again I will say, rejoice!" (Phil. 4:4).

As for human doctors, there are appropriate times to pay them a visit. If someone in your family requires a couple stitches, for example, you probably don't want to try handling that at home. Think about it—Proverbs says a merry heart does good *like a medicine.* That implies that medicine does some good.

I prefer, though, to use medicine in the form of natural remedies, which are safer than manufactured drugs. Many drugs manufactured today can be poisonous to your body and have nasty side effects. It is wise to find a physician who is judicious in what he or she prescribes. You also want to choose a physician who emphasizes nutrition and living a healthy lifestyle, not someone who concentrates on treating what ails you after the fact and typically turns to prescriptions. Any good physician knows the truth that an ounce of prevention is worth a pound of cure.

Now don't misunderstand me. Doctors and medicines are sometimes a huge blessing. When you or someone you love suffers a traumatic injury or is involved in an accident, you better believe you want a skilled physician on duty in the emergency room! Where day-to-day health is involved, however, you should apply the words of Hippocrates—the Greek physician who is considered the father of modern medicine: "Let food be thy medicine and medicine be thy food."[1]

This is the whole idea behind God-made foods. The Lord "satisfies your mouth with good things, so that your youth is renewed like the eagle's" (Ps. 103:5). You will live longer, look younger, and need less medical attention if you will "do the dos" and live according to God's perfect health plan.

TO SUPPLEMENT OR NOT TO SUPPLEMENT

Many people ask, "If I eat a balanced diet full of God-made foods, is it still necessary to take supplements?" The answer is that just to keep from being deficient in major vitamins and minerals, you would need to eat two to four fruit servings, four to six vegetable servings, and five to eleven whole grain servings every day, 365 days a year. That is not likely for most people.

In addition, eating those kinds of servings also presumes these fruits, vegetables, and whole grains are grown in non-depleted soils, which are difficult to find. United States Senate Document 264 tells us that more than 90 percent of Americans are deficient in one or more minerals because of the depleted condition of our soil.[2] So yes, taking supplements is a necessity for good health. Which ones? At a minimum, a good multivitamin and some essential fatty acids, which I discuss in the next section.

WHAT ABOUT CHOLESTEROL?

Cholesterol-managing drugs are the top-selling pharmaceuticals in this country. However, they can be as harmful as they are beneficial, depleting the body of essential nutrients. If that's the case, then what do you do about troublesome cholesterol levels? As with any medical problem, an ounce of prevention here truly is worth a pound of cure.

First, you can prevent cholesterol problems by eating nutritiously and judiciously. I mentioned earlier that a quarter cup of kidney beans and three raw carrots a day can lower bad cholesterol by as much as 30 percent. If you are on cholesterol medication, try adding those to your daily diet. The next time they check your level, your doctor may reduce your dosage or even eliminate it. If you want quick results, add sweet potatoes to your diet too. They are the best cholesterol-lowering food you can eat. Oats and garlic will also help.

Keep in mind too that eliminating every trace of fat from your diet is not the answer to lowering cholesterol. You need to understand that there are good fats and bad fats. Knowing which is vital to good health. Toxins hide in bad fats, whereas good fats benefit the body. Every cell of your body needs to take good nutrition in and get waste out. Surrounding each cell—all 100 trillion of them—is a bilipid layer that can store fat. Bad fats, which are saturated fats derived mostly from animal products, gum up that bilipid layer. Thus, your cells can't work as efficiently.

Bad fats heighten your LDL, or "bad cholesterol" level, and cause plaque on your arterial walls. Of these bad fats, the partially hydrogenated kind are horrible—probably worse than anything else! Cakes, cookies, pies, and fried foods are loaded with them. So are man-made trans fats, where oil is heated and changed to make foods thicker and creamier. For example, margarine contains trans fat. Studies have concluded that thirty thousand Americans die annually because of eating a high-fat diet. It is no wonder that in Leviticus 3:17 God commanded the Israelites to eat no fat!

Bad fats cause every cell in your body to need an "oil change." Try substituting a new oil—good fats. Make sure you get enough essential fatty acids (or "EFAs" as they are called in supplement form) to keep your cells properly lubricated. EFAs are good for your heart, brain, and immune system—every part of you. They soften your skin, boost your energy level, and help you think clearly. Taking in the proper amounts of EFAs is essential to managing cholesterol levels.

Nuts and seeds are great sources of EFAs. So are such oils as olive oil and flaxseed oil. Fish is power-packed with them—which is why two servings of fish a week can lower heart disease by 40 percent. EFAs can also be taken in supplement form. I use flaxseed and fish oils daily to get my "oil change."

When it comes to cholesterol management, "do the dos." Eat vegetables shown to reduce cholesterol, avoid processed foods high in trans and partially hydrogenated fats, eat foods high in good fats, and supplement with EFAs as needed. When you "do the dos," you can escape the bad cholesterol trap!

A SELF-CHECK HEALTH CHECK

Here is a little health check that you can do yourself. Answer these questions truthfully:

- ✓ Do you always handle stressors properly? Do you know how to four-six it?

- ✓ Do you always get enough sleep? Especially between the hours of 10:00 p.m. and 2:00 a.m.?

- ✓ Do you follow a consistent exercise program? ("Yes" means you *are* following it, not that you *plan* to follow it!)

- ✓ Do you regularly get fresh air and breathe deeply? Do you avoid smoking?

- ✓ Do you regularly get sunshine (daily if possible)?

- ✓ Are fresh fruits on your daily menu?

- ✓ Are fresh vegetables on your daily menu? (French fries don't count!)

- ✓ Are whole grains a staple of your diet? Do you typically avoid SAD—the standard American diet—of processed foods?

- ✓ When you have a choice, do you choose white meat over other meats? Do you choose lean cuts?

✓ Do you drink what you're mostly made of, water, at a rate of eight to twelve cups a day? Do you avoid alcohol, soft drinks, coffee, and other unhealthy beverages?

Did you notice that this list of questions is more like a pop quiz on my Ten Keys That Cure? How did you do? If you scored ten out of ten by answering yes every time, congratulations! That is wonderful! You are either very healthy or soon to be that way.

If you could not answer affirmatively to each question, though, take heart. You can start putting these keys into practice immediately. Start planting the seeds of better health habits today. Retakes of this health quiz are offered daily, so you can take it again tomorrow and do better than you did today!

REAPING "LIFE ABUNDANT"

Ever hear the adage "You reap what you sow"? That is true because it comes straight from the pages of Scripture: "Whatever a man sows, that he will also reap" (Gal. 6:7). Nowhere is this truer than in the area of health. I hope you have realized while reading this book that no matter what your current level of health, you can take simple, positive steps every day to reap the good health promised in God's Word.

Don't hang a long list of "don't's" on your refrigerator and make a long face every time you look at them (or try *not* to look at them). It can be discouraging to keep thinking about how far you have to go and about all the things you will have to deny yourself to get there.

Instead, hang up "Dr. Don's Be Healthy Song" lyrics and concentrate on the good things you can do that will help you gain ground every day. Be encouraged and smile when you think of how you *get to* do healthy things instead of *having to* do them. Thank God every morning for the energy to get up and get moving. If your health isn't good yet, thank God that you can at least move your big toe, and do that much until you can do more!

Four-six it whenever a problem or worry comes to mind, casting all your cares on the Lord because He cares for you. Remember that God isn't in the business of *de-stressing*, He's in the business of *no stressing*. He intends your days to be a taste of heaven on earth, something to be enjoyed instead of endured. Get outside every day and take advantage of the fresh air and sunshine He created to give you good health and pleasure.

Eat the foods God made for you, foods that fill and nourish you, keeping you healthy and strong so you can accomplish everything He has purposed for you. Make fruits and vegetables straight from the ground 50 percent of your diet. Eat satisfying, high-fiber whole grains, try a loaf of Ezekiel bread, and avoid processed foods. Choose white meat, avoid fat, and limit your consumption of other meat products. Avoid "unclean" meats, knowing God handed down the concept of clean and unclean meats in Scripture to promote health among His people. And of course, drink what you're mostly made of—water, water, and more water. Water makes your health complete.

Finally, stay in God's Word daily. God's Word tells us that He desires "that you may prosper in all things and be in health, just as your soul prospers" (3 John 2). When your mind (your soul) is renewed by the Word of God, it will transform you (Rom. 12:2), and you will have the mind of Christ in regard to your health. When you know what God's Word says about your health, you will think healthy thoughts, do healthy things, and *be* healthy—for whatever a person thinks on in his or her heart, he or she becomes (Prov. 23:7).

As John 10:10 assures us, Jesus came to give us life abundant.

When you follow God's plan in His Word, you will reap this kind of life in your health—body, soul, and spirit.

ONE MORE KIND OF WATER

Before concluding this chapter, I want to suggest one more kind of water to you. "Whoever takes a drink of the water that I will give him shall never, no never, be thirsty again," Jesus said to the woman at the well. "But the water that I will give him shall become a spring of water welling up (flowing, bubbling) [continually] within him unto (into, for) eternal life" (John 4:14, AMP).

If you feel a thirsting inside you that is not physical and an intense longing for something more to life—though you're not quite sure what—you may be spiritually dehydrated. You need a drink of the living water Jesus was talking about. A relationship with God, your heavenly Father and Creator, will satisfy this intense inner thirst. If you don't know Him yet, you can come into His family today by accepting His Son, Jesus, as your Lord and Savior. The Bible promises that "whosoever shall call upon the name of the Lord shall be saved" (Rom. 10:13, KJV). That "whosoever" means *you*, no matter who you are, where you've been, or what you've done. If anyone, including *you*, will "confess with your mouth the Lord Jesus and believe in your heart that God has raised Him from the dead, you will be saved" (Rom. 10:9).

Simply pray the following prayer aloud with all your heart:

O God, I come to You in Jesus's name. I believe that Jesus died on the cross, shed His blood for me, and paid for my sins. I believe He rose again and gave me the gift of eternal life, and I receive Him as Lord of my life. Jesus, I am Yours now and forever. I know You have a plan and a purpose for my life, and I believe You want me healthy and whole, spirit, soul, and body, so that I can serve You all my days. I thank You for giving me the living water and for hearing my prayer. I give you my life from this day forward. In Jesus's name, amen.

Welcome to the family of God and to the river of life and health you will find in knowing Him! The Bible promises that "His divine power has given to us all things that pertain to life and godliness, through the knowledge of Him who called us by glory and virtue" (2 Pet. 1:3). Enjoying good biblical health certainly pertains to life and godliness! With that precious promise in mind, let's go out and live for God in great biblical health, blessing others as He has blessed us all along the way.

DR. DON'S EASY REFERENCE GUIDE FOR COMMON HEALTH PROBLEMS

CHAPTER 12

DR. DON'S EASY REFERENCE GUIDE FOR COMMON HEALTH PROBLEMS

ACHIEVING IDEAL WEIGHT: *LEAN* ON THE LORD

Do you want to lose weight? LEAN on the Lord. Don't skip meals. Instead, show your gratitude for the nourishment He provides by eating slowly, savoring each bite. Did you know it takes your stomach twenty minutes to tell your brain you are full? In addition to appreciating the food God provides you, eat only when you are hungry—physically hungry. Avoid the temptation to use food as a treatment for depression, anxiety, or stress—or, as so many in this modern age, as a source of entertainment. LEANing includes:

L - liquids

If you want to lose weight, drinking plenty of water is essential and important for good health. Water constitutes up to 70 percent of your body tissues, 80 percent of brain tissues, and 90 percent of blood. It detoxifies you, cleanses you, and lubricates your very cells. Drinking eight to twelve glasses a day will help you lose weight. Start your day with water. Drink a full glass an hour before meals. Feeling hungry? Maybe you're thirsty! Fill up on a glass of no-calorie water and see if you can wait a while longer before eating.

E - exercise

Exercise does more than burn fat and calories. It gives you more energy and releases endorphins—those "feel-good" brain chemicals. Exercise also increases the oxygen-carrying capacity of cells throughout your body, boosting your immune system while building your muscle. And muscle is your best friend in weight loss. After meals, engage in light exercise to boost your metabolism. Make a decision to start exercising *now*—even if you are relaxing in your recliner.

A - add and avoid

- Add high-fiber, complex carbohydrate foods to your diet—such as raw fruits, raw vegetables, and 100 percent whole-grain breads and pastas.

- Add good proteins: legumes, egg whites, lean meats, and grilled fish.

- Add more fresh foods, prepared from scratch.

- Avoid trans fats, saturated fats, hydrogenated oils, and fractionated oils. These build fat that your body doesn't know how to burn.

- Avoid sugar, especially high-fructose corn syrup—a highly processed monster that builds stubborn belly fat.

- Avoid fast foods and convenience foods that serve up bad fats, sugar, and additives instead of God-given natural nutrients.

N - nutrients

If you are working hard, drinking water, eating right, and exercising—you still need a boost! Add a good multivitamin with B vitamins, chromium, and vanadium.

ADHD: DIET OR DRUGS?

Are you or your child...

- Hyperactive, fidgety, and unable to sit still?

- Impulsive and unable to finish what you started?

- Unable to pay attention, making careless mistakes?

If you are human, you probably can answer yes to all these questions—depending on what's going on in your life at the moment. Or you may have been diagnosed with ADHD, which I call a non-disease. It was created to describe symptoms that could indicate food allergies, an overstressed lifestyle, anxiety, depression, lead poisoning, or a learning disability.

I define ADHD as simple incompatibility between a person and his or her environment. Lifestyle changes, such as changing jobs, finding alternative education, or improving your diet, can often solve the problem.

To address dietary problems, eat real food, not processed: fresh fruits and vegetables, whole grains, and "brain" foods. Include flax-seed oil for essential fatty acids and fish oil or wild-caught fish for docosahexaenoic acids (DHA) and eicosapentaenoic acids (EPA). Support serotonin production with turkey, sunflower seeds, and bananas. Also, use the pulse test (which checks your pulse rate; you can find more information online) or an elimination diet to rule out food allergies. Common triggers for food allergies are sugar, cow's milk, wheat, yeast, corn, eggs, or chocolate.

Also, supplement your diet with a high-quality multivitamin/ mineral (B vitamins, calcium, zinc, magnesium, and chromium are essential) and a glyconutrient source. This is a supplement containing a blend of simple sugars.

Detoxify. A high-fiber diet and supplements will start the process. Reinforce with fasting, and consult your health care provider to see if parasite control night be needed. Cook from scratch and avoid such toxins as artificial colors, flavors, additives, and preservatives. Be aware that poor dietary absorption of naturally chelating nutrients can cause heavy metal toxicity.

Avoid chemical treatments. On February 9, 2006, a FDA advisory panel voted to recommend adding its strongest warning label—a "black box" label—for Ritalin, Adderall, Focalin, Methylin, Metadate, Concerta, and other medications used to treat ADHD/ADD.[1]

Start your day with this "Brain Shake":

1 scoop of soy protein powder
1 scoop of green powder
2 Tbsp. ground flaxseed
1 banana
½ cup soy milk
½ cup orange juice (not from concentrate)

Blend and enjoy a brain happy day!

ALKALIZE YOUR DIET AND KISS THE FAT GOOD-BYE

Do you know your pH? Probably not. If you eat like most Americans, chances are your pH level will err on the acidic side. Processed foods, fast foods, and packaged foods all contribute to acidifying your body chemistry. Even naturally alkaline foods become acidic during industrialized food processing. Other acidifying agents are caffeine, alcohol, and antibiotics. Stress and inactivity also cause acidity to rise.

An acidic body environment causes all kinds of mischief, including weight gain and obesity. You see, the body responds to acidic molecules by wrapping them in tough-to-lose fat. It stores them safely away from the heart—on the buttocks, abdomen, and thighs. Acidic pH also causes increased blood sugar, another factor in weight gain.

Eat slimming alkaline foods!

Most fruits and vegetables, especially greens, are alkaline. Exceptions are cranberries and beans. You may wonder how acidic citrus fruits can be considered alkaline; the digestive process turns the alkaline in your body.

Very high alkaline foods

- Bananas

- Chocolate

- Figs

- Orange juice

- Potatoes

- Spinach

- Watermelon

- Dandelion greens

Avoid processed foods!

Just because a food is naturally high in acid content does not automatically mean it is unhealthy. Including naturally acidic foods in fresh, made-from-scratch recipes probably won't hurt you a bit. Problems such as weight gain arise when your diet does not include alkaline foods, instead relying on processed, packaged, and fast foods. Processing turns naturally alkaline food acidic.

How processed foods impact your pH

Human blood pH should be slightly alkaline (7.35 to 7.45). A reading below or above this range means symptoms and disease. If blood pH moves below 6.8 or above 7.8, cells stop functioning and the body dies. When this balance is compromised, many problems can occur. Therefore, the body continually strives to balance pH.

An imbalanced diet high in acidic-producing foods, such as animal protein, sugar, caffeine, and processed foods, puts pressure on the body's regulating systems that maintain pH neutrality. The extra buffering required can deplete the body of alkaline minerals, such as sodium, potassium, magnesium, and calcium. This makes you prone to chronic and degenerative disease. Minerals are borrowed from vital organs and bones to buffer (neutralize) the acid and safely remove it from the body. Because of this strain, the body can suffer severe and prolonged damage. Yet the condition may go undetected for years.

It's what you eat, not how much you eat

Weight gain can have as much to do with what you eat as how much you eat. Some overweight people can eat as many carbohydrates as they desire. As long as they are foods with a low-glycemic index, these people still lose weight. These are whole, fresh, fiber-rich foods that are minimally processed and low in sugars and fats, such as non-starchy vegetables, fresh fruits, beans and peas, 100 percent whole grains, nuts, and dairy products.

Examples of low-glycemic foods include black beans, broccoli, cherries, leafy vegetables, milk, peanuts and peanut butter, pears, plums, soybeans, tomatoes, wild rice, yogurt, and whole grains.

Among moderately low-glycemic foods are apples, garbanzo beans (chickpeas), ice cream, navy beans, oranges, peas, pinto beans, and potato chips. On the moderately high side are bananas, candy bars, potatoes, white pita bread, oat, oat bread, raisins, carrots, brown rice, and kidney beans.

Include exercise!

If you do not exercise, weight loss is tougher. If you live a sedentary life, your metabolism may have dropped to "starvation mode." If you reduce what you eat enough to lose weight with such low metabolism, you will not be able to get all the nutrients you need.

So while you get in the alkaline food habit, get in the exercise habit too!

Acidosis puts you at risk

Acidosis can lead to many health problems in addition to weight gain. Acidosis decreases your ability to absorb nutrients, impairs cellular energy production and repair, makes your body unable to excrete certain toxins, and increases your susceptibility to fatigue and illness.

Acidosis can cause:

- Cardiovascular damage

- Diabetes

- Gastritis, bladder and kidney problems

- Osteoporosis, joint and muscle pain

- Slow digestion and elimination

- Yeast/fungal overgrowth

- Depression and stress

- Headaches, dental and eye problems, mouth ulcers, and cracked lips

- Unhealthy hair, skin, and nails

ALLERGIES & SWEETS: SUGAR IS NOTHING TO SNEEZE AT

A spoonful of sugar may help the medicine go down. But if you eat much more than that, sugar can make you sick—especially if you have allergies. Sugar can provoke an inflammatory response that is identical to an allergic immune response. If you already have allergies, you may well double your misery.

Why, you may ask? For one, because sugar suppresses your immune system. If you eat mounds of sugar, you are not only more likely to experience an allergic event, but you will also be less able to fight off viruses and bacterial infections. If that weren't bad enough, sugar can cause your cells to swell and aggravate allergic swelling you are already experiencing if you have an allergy.

Where is it hiding?

You won't be surprised to know that candy, ice cream, cookies, pastries, and sweet desserts have a lot of sugar. But sugar hides in numerous other foods. Did you know that a can of soda pop has about 12 teaspoons of sugar in it? Fruit juices often have a high sugar content as well, which is why it is better to get servings from a piece of fresh fruit, not a glass of processed juice.

Just because its makers tout a product as "natural" and "healthy" does not make it so. Take a closer look at the facts on the nutrition label (most often on a side panel). Most granola bars, flavored yogurts, yogurt smoothies, trail mixes, and commercial whole-grain cereals are packed with sugar.

The USDA requires manufacturers to list label ingredients in order of quantity. If the first ingredient is sugar, there is more sugar in the product than anything else. Manufacturers think they can trick you by using many different types of sugar. That way they don't have to list any of them first. Fructose, lactose, and dextrose are all types of sugar, as indicated by the -ose suffix. So are corn syrup, sorbitol, mannitol, maltitol, and xylitol. So the granola bar that lists whole grain as its first ingredient and follows with a list of three or four of these kinds of sugars may well be as sweet as cotton candy.

Sugar also hides in high-glycemic carbs such as potato chips and white bread. These carbs quickly convert to sugar in your body.

Sweet seduction

Allopathic doctors do not recognize sugar as an allergen. The rationale is that since our body breaks down our foods into glucose (blood sugar), how in the world could one be allergic to it? However, naturopathic doctors, informed nutritionists, and alternative health practitioners have been warning us about the dangers of sugar for decades.

While sugar won't cause a response on a standard allergy test, too much sugar (or high-glycemic carbs) causes an inflammatory response identical to the immune response. Why? Excess sugar interferes with the absorption of vitamins and minerals crucial to healthy immune response, makes mayhem with your metabolism, and disables your neurotransmitters. The energy rush and insulin spike that you get from sugar creates an imbalanced body chemistry.

Artificial sweeteners are not the answer

Many people kicking the sugar habit turn to NutraSweet (aspartame), Splenda (sucralose), or Sweet 'N Low (saccharin). All can pose disastrous side effects. Aspartame has a list of side effects as long as your arm, including blindness, hearing impairment, seizures, depression, irritability, hives, menstrual irregularities, hair loss, and gradual weight gain. Splenda users have reported bladder pain, irritable bowel syndrome, extreme abdominal cramping, symptoms mimicking stroke and heart attack, panic attacks, painful skin rashes, and life-threatening anaphylactic shock. Saccharin causes cancer.

More sugar dangers

If you have allergies, that's one good reason to reduce the amount of sugar in your diet. If you don't have allergies, too much sugar can still do you harm.

Other sugar facts

- Sugar places major demands on your digestive system and interferes with absorption of crucial vitamins and minerals.

- Sugar wreaks havoc on your metabolism, making it difficult for you to absorb the healthy foods you are eating.

- Sugar depletes valuable neurotransmitters that help you think clearly. Confusion, forgetfulness, ADHD, and depression are symptoms that can occur as much as two days after eating sugar.

- The energy rush and insulin spike that you get from sugar creates an imbalance in your body chemistry. This can lead to weight gain, insulin resistance, and loss of appetite control.

- Muscle cramping, PMS, joint pain, and fatigue are other common symptoms of sugar sensitivity.

Despite these alarming affects, reducing the amount of sugar you eat can be a challenge. This is because of a basic biological fact: the more you eat, the more you want! Those who want to cut down can start by reading labels carefully so you can avoid hidden sugars. Skip sugary juices and soft drinks—opt instead for a glass of water with a twist of lemon. Because sugar hides in so many things (like the ketchup most people dip their fries in), avoid fast foods, and cook from scratch when you can.

When that inevitable sugar craving raises its ugly head, try a piece of fruit or cheese. If you must give in, have a cup of herbal tea with a half-teaspoon of honey. Honey is twice as sweet as sugar and impacts blood sugar levels less dramatically. Sugar dulls your sensitivity to the natural sugars in fruit. After you kick your sugar habit, fruit may taste better than ever. The more fruit you eat, the better!

Building resistance to allergies is all about building better overall health. Your health is what you eat. Note: Organic foods do not contain the preservatives and colorings that aggravate hay fever, allergic rhinitis, and other allergies.

Some helpful guidelines

1. Select organic fruit and vegetables whenever possible. Wash or peel nonorganic produce.

2. Choose fruits and vegetables in season. This limits your exposure to the chemicals used to delay ripening, prolong shelf-life, preserve color, and so on.

3. Eat whole grains. They carry a lower glycemic load (convert to sugar slower) and give you more vitamins, minerals, and protein.

4. Supplement your diet with antioxidant nutrients: vitamins A, C, and E, and the minerals zinc and selenium, since detoxifying from many pesticides requires these nutrients.

5. Eliminate milk and other dairy products (especially if they are not organic) from your diet. In addition, know your producer! The USDA allows some so-called organic factory farms to raise dairy cattle that are given feed contaminated with pesticides, hormones, and antibiotics as long as the animals are on an organic diet when they start giving milk.

ALZHEIMER'S DISEASE: STRATEGIES TO REMEMBER

Every sixty-nine seconds, another American develops Alzheimer's disease.[2] Currently, 5.4 million Americans have the disease—5.2 million of these are age sixty-five and older.[3] By 2050 the number of

Americans with Alzheimer's will rise to 16 million.[4] What is causing this epidemic of dementia?

Many experts agree that the American lifestyle and diet are contributing factors. So too are certain prescription medications. For example, the drug Detrol—prescribed for overactive bladder and incontinence—causes dementia that is often misdiagnosed as Alzheimer's disease. (The "disease" labeled overactive bladder is really no disease at all. The condition was invented by Detrol's manufacturer to boost sales![5])

In addition, prescription drugs used to treat Alzheimer's provide little help or hope. The blockbuster drug Aricept brings its makers nearly $2 billion a year in sales but does little for the patients taking it ($1,500 a year per patient). Aricept's common side effects include vomiting, dizziness, and insomnia. Physicians often prescribe antidepressants, tranquilizers, and anti-psychotic medications to patients with Alzheimer's. These too do very little to ameliorate their condition while exposing patients to a wide range of potentially dangerous side effects.

Avoiding Alzheimer's

Ensuring good overall health is the best way to avoid Alzheimer's. Eat wholesome, God-made foods such as fruits, vegetables, whole grains, and healthy fats—almonds, walnuts, and fish oils found in salmon and other cold-water fish. People who eat fish one time a week reduce their risk of getting Alzheimer's by 50 percent. Half of your brain is fat. Eating bad fats can hurt your brain; eating good fats can help it. This is why I say to go easy on red meat; it has too much bad fat.

While eating good foods, phase out fast foods and prepared substances with long lists of chemical ingredients or additives. Drinking plenty of water every day also helps brain function. Did you know that most children's bodies are 75 percent water while most elderly folks are only 50 percent? Stay hydrated, and you may age more slowly.

Exercise your brain and your body! Physical exercise helps balance your blood sugar. High blood sugar and insulin levels, as well as diabetes, are associated with increased risk of Alzheimer's disease. No matter what your age, it is never too late to start exercising. Try walking or, if you have arthritis, water aerobics. Tai chi is another excellent exercise for older adults.

Brain exercises

For starters, one of the best ways you can exercise your brain is to turn off the TV and engage in the real world. In addition, try:

- Reading

- Doing brain games such as crossword puzzles, Sudoku, or picture puzzles

- Playing chess, cards, dominoes, or other board games that require mental focus

Supplementation

Ask your alternative health care provider for proper dosages of the following supplements, which have been proven to help prevent Alzheimer's disease:

- Fish oil capsules

- Vitamin E

- Vitamin C

- B vitamins, especially folic acid

- Beta-carotene

- NAC (N-acetylcysteine)

- ALA (alpha lipoic acid)

- ALC (acetyl-L-carnitine)

- CoQ_{10} (coenzyme Q_{10})

In addition, use curry and turmeric spices to flavor your favorite home-cooked dishes. Both have proven brain health benefits.

In conclusion

If you or someone you love has been diagnosed with Alzheimer's disease, take these positive steps:

- Build brain power through exercise, good nutrition, and supplementation.

- Investigate prescription medications. Their side effects might be the real culprit in dementia.

- Find support. Alzheimer's devastates relationships and gobbles up financial resources. Find friends at church or a support group through your local Alzheimer's organization to help you cope. As doctors suggest expensive drug therapies, be aware that these will not cure Alzheimer's and may not even help slow its progression. If the medication isn't working, don't be afraid to terminate its use.

ASTHMA: FOODS THAT
SOOTHE, FOODS TO AVOID

Do you have asthma? Does your child have asthma? Then you have experienced the terror and irritation that happens when airways become so sensitive and swollen that you cough, wheeze, and struggle to catch your breath. Asthma symptoms can be triggered by exercise; cold air; such toxins as allergens, pollutants, and viruses; and food.

Detoxify your world

We live in a toxic world. The air we breathe contains pollutants and viruses. The water we drink may have chlorine, fluoride, and other decontaminants. While our bodies work hard to eliminate these toxins from our systems, sometimes there are just too many. You reach the point where that last toxic straw breaks your immune system's back. If you are like twenty million other Americans, your body reacts with an asthma attack.

The first step to having fewer asthma attacks is to avoid toxins. I realize this may be easier said than done. However, do your best to avoid situations and environments where you will encounter allergens that trigger your attacks. During pollen seasons or on ozone action days, stay indoors or wear a protective mask. Other steps you can take:

- In your home try to keep allergens, dust, and dust mites at bay.

- Use air filtration and houseplants to cleanse indoor air. Don't forget to throw the windows open now and then to freshen the air, as well.

- Wash your bedding in hot water every week.

- Brush your pets daily to reduce the amount of dander floating about.

- Use nontoxic, "green" cleaning products—or good old baking soda and vinegar—in your home. Avoid commercial air fresheners.

- Paint your walls with low-VOC-rating paints, and avoid those plastics and furnishings that emit chemical gases.

Detoxify your body

For starters, drink eight to twelve glasses of *pure* water every day. Your best water source may well be your own tap—provided you have attached a filtration system that specifically filters out fluoride and other contaminants. Plastic water bottles not only overburden our landfills, but they also emit small amounts of toxins into the water they hold.

Cleansing the colon can also help detoxify your body. An easy and practical way to keep your colon clean is to eat more high-fiber foods (whole grains, fresh fruits, and raw vegetables) while avoiding processed foods and sugar.

Better brEAThing

Did you know food allergies are a major trigger for asthma attacks? The standard American diet of refined, packaged, additive-ridden processed foods aggravates asthma. These foods lack the nutrients you need to build your health—and contain unhealthy food additives.

The following chart details common additives in everyday foods that aggravate asthma.

Calcium benzoate	In drinks, low-sugar products, cereals, meats	Aggravates hay fever, hives, and asthma
Calcium sulphite	Many foods	Aggravates bronchial problems, asthma, and cardiovascular problems
Sodium metabisulphite	Many foods	Provokes life-threatening asthma
Sulphur dioxide	Many foods	Causes bronchial problems in those with asthma or low blood pressure
Brilliant Black BN Allura RedAC Ponceau 4R, Cochineal, Red A Sunset Yellow FCF, Orange Yellow S Tartrazine	Many foods	Aggravates asthma symptoms

In a clinical study of children with life-threatening asthma, more than 50 percent were found to have food allergies—such as to peanuts—compared to only 10 percent in the control group.[6] This posed the possibility that life-threatening asthma attacks are triggered by food allergies.

Other foods that commonly cause food allergies are cow's milk, wheat, yeast, eggs, sugar, soy, corn, and chocolate. Pulse testing or an elimination diet can help you determine which foods cause you or your child to have an asthma attack.

Foods that relieve and prevent asthma

When your body is well nourished, your immune system has the natural power it needs to handle toxins and allergens. These foods have been proven to help your immune system relieve and prevent asthma attacks:

- Generous amounts of fresh organic fruits and vegetables

- 100 percent whole grains: breads, cereal, pasta, and crackers

- Cold-water fish: cod, salmon, mackerel, halibut, salmon, tuna, sardines, and herring

- Extra-virgin olive oil

- Flaxseeds or flaxseed oil

- Herbal spices: rosemary, ginger, and turmeric

Picture a salad of mixed greens with olive oil and balsamic vinegar accompanying a juicy, pink salmon steak baked with fresh rosemary and served on a plate of tender steamed vegetables and some sweet, ripe fruit. A satisfying meal like this is ideal if you have asthma.

In addition, consider a vegetarian diet. Did you know that people who embark on a vegetarian diet usually relieve their allergy symptoms within twelve months?

Why organic?

Eating organic foods will help you avoid the food additives that trigger asthma as well as the pesticide residues that can also trigger asthma attacks. In fact, for asthma sufferers, eating organic can be a matter of life and breath.

Organic is important because of conventionally harvested goods, between 89 and 99 percent of these fresh fruits, grains, and vegetables are sprayed with pesticides. In random testing, some fruits—particularly strawberries, raspberries, grapes, and tomatoes—had residues of at least six different pesticides! Carrots and lettuce were found to have pesticide residue levels up to twenty-five times higher than acceptable USDA limits. Pesticides are also used to treat animal feed, which contaminates most meat, milk, and dairy products.

Three basic guidelines with food:

1. Select organic fruit and vegetables whenever possible. Wash or peel nonorganic produce.

2. Choose fruits and vegetables in season. This means that your exposure to the chemicals used to delay ripening, prolong shelf life, preserve color, and so on will be limited.

3. Eliminate milk and other dairy products, especially if they are not organic. Know your producer! As I stated earlier, the USDA allows some so-called organic factory farms to raise dairy cattle on pesticide-contaminated feed, hormones, and antibiotics—as long as the animals are on an organic diet when they begin giving milk.

Help your foods help your body

Because of the ways modern foods are processed and delivered, they often lose the essential phytonutrients (bioactive, plant-derived compounds) needed to maintain health. This is why it is important to supplement your diet with quality-grade nutraceutical products, targeted to each individual's health needs. If you or someone you love has asthma, consider supplementation.

As a preventive measure, take a good, natural (not synthetic) multivitamin that provides generous quantities of vitamin A, B_6, B_{12}, C, and E; the minerals zinc, magnesium, and selenium; antioxidants; and bioflavanoids. In addition, aloe vera and garlic can help balance and fortify the immune system, while flax or fish oil can reduce the inflammatory-allergic response.

BLADDER INFECTIONS: COMMONSENSE CARE

Affecting more women than men, bladder infections cause pain, discomfort, and inconvenience. If left untreated, they can become more serious infections that migrate into the kidneys. Bladder infections are common among women today for a variety of reasons.

What you eat and drink

If evil scientists searched for a way to cause an epidemic of bladder infections in a population, they would have to look no further than the standard American diet. Sugar, refined carbohydrates (which convert to sugar in the body), and the hosts of chemical additives all set the bladder up for infection. Both regular and diet soda pop promote bladder infection. Plus, when it comes to soda pop, you introduce two more badder-bladder factors: caffeine and sodium benzoate. Both act as diuretics, drying up your poor bladder so it has no choice but to strike back.

If you want to quit having constant bladder infections, kick the sugar habit. Drink pure water in place of soda pop, sugary juices, or artificially sweetened beverages. Plus, change your carb intake to 100 percent whole-grain breads and pastas.

What you don't drink

Most of us don't drink enough water—for adults, that means eight to twelve 8-ounce glasses a day.

What you wear

Another enemy of a woman's bladder is constrictive clothing made of synthetic fabrics. Tight, polyester pants and nylon pantyhose restrict air flow and encourage the growth of bacteria. These bacteria can back up into the bladder through the urethra. Thong underwear also encourages this kind of contamination. If possible, wear looser pants or skirts, cotton underwear, and avoid pantyhose.

Hygiene

From the time they are toddlers, girls should be taught to wipe their bottoms from front to back after bowel movements. Bacteria from bowel movements can be introduced into the bladder via the urethral opening when girls wipe back to front. Bubble bath has also been implicated as a cause of bladder infections, especially among young girls.

If you have a bladder infection, these tips may help clear it up more quickly:

- Empty your bladder often; don't "hold it."

- Empty your bladder before and after intercourse.

- Drink a glass of water every waking hour.

- Eat fresh parsley and celery to increase urine flow.

- Cranberry juice makes bladder walls slippery (a good thing). However, try to find unsweetened cranberry juice or herbal cranberry tea, since sugar and artificial sweeteners can worsen your condition.

- Avoid all sugar, alcohol, carbonated drinks, chocolate, caffeine, and processed foods.

- Alkalize your urine by taking a half teaspoon of baking soda in a glass of water, twice a day.

- Add a good source of L. acidophilus—available in many yogurts or in pill or powder form—to your diet.

- The herb uva ursi acts as a natural diuretic to get infection out. Aloe vera juice (1 to 3 ounces daily) and echinacea can boost your immune system's response.

- Supplement with a high-quality multivitamin and mineral formula daily.

CANCER AND SELF-CARE

If you or a loved one has been diagnosed with cancer, you may feel like life is spinning out of control. You are probably shuffling to countless doctor's appointments, undergoing a host of unfamiliar procedures, and ingesting medications with names that are tough to pronounce. You may feel like a stranger in a strange land, forced to learn a new language. While the temptation may be to give up and give yourself over to your medical team, remember that no one cares about your condition more than you do. By taking responsibility for your own health care, researching alternatives, and taking some basic steps in self-care, you will increase your chances of beating cancer and getting your life back.

Basic lifestyle guidelines

If you were eating a good, healthy, natural, organic diet before your diagnosis of cancer, now is no time to abandon it. If not, now is the time to start. Many cancer patients have discovered that switching their nutritional intake makes a huge difference in their outcome and quality of life. Follow these basics in your daily routine:

- Eat whole, raw foods as often as possible: organically grown fruits, vegetables, and whole grains.

- Drink eight glasses of pure, filtered water every day.

- Include a tablespoon of flaxseed oil daily for essential fatty acids (EFAs).

- Take a natural vitamin-mineral supplement.

In addition, it will be helpful to observe a three-to-five-day juice fast once every six months. For three days drink only freshly juiced organic vegetables and fruits, along with plenty of pure, filtered water.

While eating a healthy diet, say "absolutely not" to the following:

- Fried foods

- Meat and dairy products

- Alcohol and smoking

- Artificial food colorings or flavorings and preservatives

- Processed foods, which are strictly forbidden. Eat nothing that says enriched, fortified, or bleached on the label or has strange ingredients that you can't identify.

Detoxify

Detoxification is a natural function addressed by many of your body's systems. However, sometimes the toxic overload becomes too much for the body to handle. Both the causes—and some of the "cures" traditional medicine offers—of your cancer may build up toxins in your body. Routine detoxification supports your body in its fight to rid you of substances and by-products that impair your health (specifically the immune system).

For starters, clean and replenish your GI tract. More than one-half of the immune system operates from here. In addition:

- For normal colon function, use an herbal-fiber bowel restorer to encourage at least two bowel movements daily.

- Supplement with digestive enzymes and probiotics, e.g., acidophilus.

- Lose excess fat, since this is where toxins hide.

- Support liver and kidney function with the herb milk thistle and greens.

Fortify

When it comes to your immune system, cancer and its treatments pack a wallop. You do not have to sit back and let your immune system deteriorate. Instead, you can take steps to strengthen it by doing the following:

- Learn to relax. Stress is the immune system's number one enemy. Walk every day, if you can. Connect with nature. Schedule a regular therapeutic massage.

- Get plenty of rest, exercise, sunshine, and fresh air.

- Eat properly: fruits vegetables, whole grains, water.

- Exercise consistently to move immune fluids around your body. I generally recommend thirty-minute sessions, three to five times a week. Brisk walking is great exercise!

- Increase antioxidant levels with four glasses of green tea per day. Or juice with green powder, wheatgrass, or barley grass.

If you are undergoing chemotherapy, also:

- Take a balanced multiple vitamin/mineral supplement. This is of utmost importance!

- Avoid meat and dairy products. Concentrate on raw fruits and vegetables (juicing is best), whole grains, and natural, non-processed foods. Dietary changes are a must!

- Get plenty of rest.

- Drinking aloe juice daily will help rebuild your immune system. Get plenty of fluids, especially pure, filtered water.

- Eat ten raw almonds a day. Almonds contain an important ingredient that is toxic to cancer cells but not to normal ones. This also applies to other nuts and seeds, especially apricot seeds.

Science and supplementation

I would like to recommend two books for people choosing cancer treatments. Both are by Ralph W. Moss, PhD. One is titled *Questioning Chemotherapy*; the other is called *The Cancer Industry.* The misconception that nutrients will interfere with chemotherapy has been clearly disproven in the literature. When a person undergoes chemotherapy or radiation, he or she is generating an enormous amount of toxic metabolites released from dying cells. To detoxify these poisons and remove them from the body requires an enormous amount of extra vitamins and minerals.

Any physician who recommends not using nutritional remedies during cancer treatment is simply uninformed. The immune system is still battling cancer even in—and especially during—chemotherapy, radiation, and surgery. If there was ever a time you need your immune system to be strengthened, this would be the time. To avoid at least using a multiple vitamin and mineral supplement daily is not wise.

Yet some physicians still operate under the false notion that supplements can interfere with chemotherapy. They have a misguided belief that chemotherapy kills cancer by inflicting oxidative, free-radical damage.

In reality, not only does supplement use during chemotherapy have no downside, but it has tremendous benefits. Chemotherapy compromises the immune system and is often associated with extreme malnutrition. Supplements address both of these potentially dangerous side effects.

Christ is the "cancer answer"

Yes, you can overcome even cancer cells! You simply need to equip your immune system with the tools it needs to wage war against cancer and other diseases—and win. Terrible fear grips most people when they hear the word *cancer*, but cancer is not the "big C" word, Christ Jesus is! He's the "cancer answer."

If you have been diagnosed with cancer or another life-threatening or debilitating illness, your body may have lost a battle, but that doesn't mean you've lost the war. You can begin turning the tide of battle today. Start with believing God's Word when it says that "by His stripes we are healed" (Isa. 53:5). Search Scripture for other passages that promise healing and wholeness for the children of God (there are many), and speak them over your life daily. Then take a closer look at how God designed your immune system.

Did you know the average person's body experiences two thousand cancerous changes *daily*? A cancer cell is one that starts dividing uncontrollably, which happens two thousand times a day—in everyone. Did you know most people develop about half a dozen tumors in their lifetimes, which doctors could detect if they examined the right place at the right time? Yet not everyone gets diagnosed with cancer or undergoes cancer treatment six times in their lives. Why not? Because the immune system is specifically designed to stop the spread of cancer and other diseases. Sickness is no match for strong immune systems in detoxified bodies!

"T4 killer cells," or the white blood cells in the immune system, rid people's bodies of cancerous cells and malicious invaders such as viruses and bacteria. T4 cells resemble the old video game Pac-Man, where the yellow hero goes around gobbling up everything in his path. That is a picture of God's chemotherapy and radiation treatment happening daily in each of us.

If your body hasn't stayed on top of cancerous changes or hasn't successfully warded off other illnesses, it is time to confess the Word of God for healing and give your body some new tools to use in waging war on this dreaded disease.

CHRONIC FATIGUE AND FIBROMYALGIA: SYNDROMES WITH SOLUTIONS

More than eight hundred thousand people in the United States suffer with the debilitating symptoms of chronic fatigue syndrome (CFS). Another five million have been diagnosed with fibromyalgia syndrome (FMS). If you have either, you may experience:

- Loss of healthful, deep sleep patterns

- Hormonal imbalances

- Lingering flu symptoms

- Irritable bowel syndrome

- Headaches, facial and body pain

- Heightened sensitivity to light, noise, touch, and odors

- Exhaustion

- Swelling and tenderness in your lymph glands

Sharing a common cause?

Many experts contend that CFS and FMS share more than some common symptoms. These conditions may also share a common cause—and in fact be a progression of the same disorder. Dr. Derek Enlander, a physician treating CFS and FMS patients in New York City and faculty member at Mount Sinai Medical Center, believes that CFS and FMS are related illnesses. He says that whatever initiates an illness directly affects the immune system into an "up-regulated" or deregulated condition; this means the body, which is always trying to heal itself and return to a natural balance, is constantly adjusting to find that balance.

In years past CFS and FMS were thought to be imaginary illnesses; their symptoms seemed to have no logical explanation, and most patients experiencing the conditions were women. Though now recognized by the medical community, hard facts as to their cause and treatment are still few and far between. However, recent research has uncovered some amazing discoveries.

Mike O' Who?

Doctors discovered that a specific mycoplasma (a genus of bacteria that lack a cell wall) represented a common cause of CFS and FMS. This research was conducted by Dr. Garth Nicolson, chief scientific officer and research professor with the Institute for Molecular Medicine, and co-researchers Dr. Nancy L. Nicolson and Dr. Darryl See.[7]

Mycoplasmas are the smallest self-replicating organisms known to science. Hundreds of types of mycoplasmas can be found in plants, insects, and animals, but only a few in the human body. While not all mycoplasmas cause disease, some do—for example, *M. pneumoniae* causes walking pneumonia.

According to Dr. Nicolson, once in the cell, these bacteria steal lipids (fats) like cholesterol from the mitochondria, the components of a cell that produces energy. This makes the mitochondria "leaky," and they lose electrons, he says—similar to a battery with no insulation running down. The doctor says this may be why patients with this condition are almost always fatigued. Since their cellular batteries are low, fewer high energy molecules are available, meaning they are exhausted at the cellular level.[8]

These researchers agree that long-term antimicrobials should be initiated to treat mycoplasmal infections. They also recommend boosting the immune system and supplementing with essential nutrients and vitamins. Dr. See says that they always seek to use the least toxic approaches in working with pathologies, which is why they use numerous natural products. Examples include probiotics and undenatured whey protein isolates for supporting the GI tract. This combination helps prevent overgrowth of undesirable microorganisms.[9]

CFS and FMS may share other common causes

Those with these conditions often have lower-than-normal serotonin levels. Hence, they have problems sleeping. Hypothyroidism (underactive thyroid) may also play a role. Chronic yeast overgrowth (*Candida albicans*) has also been cited as a culprit. Since CFS and FMS sufferers are more prone to infections, doctors may frequently prescribe sufferers antibiotics. However, these stimulate yeast overgrowth, and a vicious cycle begins.

Treating any of these causes individually may help relieve your symptoms. Select herbs and foods that will help bring your body back into balance. Raw whole foods are best, especially vegetables. Good nutrition is a must. Fast foods and processed foods are stripped of their original nutrients—nutrients vital to health.

Drug dangers

If you suffer with CFS or FMS, chances are your doctor has prescribed medications to help you deal with your symptoms. Be aware that both over-the-counter and prescription medications may cause you to experience potentially dangerous and painful side effects:

- Aspirin, ibuprofen (Motrin, Advil, Nuprin, Rufin), and naproxen (Aleve, Naprosyn, Naprelan, Anaprox) may trigger gastrointestinal problems, ulcers, internal

DO THIS AND LIVE HEALTHY

bleeding, increased blood pressure, dizziness, tinnitus, headaches, rashes, and depression.

- Celebrex, Vioxx, and Bextra can increase risk of heart attack, adversely affect digestion and kidney function, and increase blood pressure. Meanwhile, other anti-inflammatories, such as meloxicam (Mobic), may increase risk of heart attack, adversely affect kidney function, and increase blood pressure.

- Tricyclic antidepressants can cause dry mouth, restlessness, reduced sexual drive, increased heart rate, constipation, and possible death by overdose.

- Cortisol, steroidal hormone supplements, and hydrocortisone can cause insomnia, weight gain, and suppressed adrenal gland function.

CHOLESTEROL: FINDING BALANCE

Regardless of what you have heard elsewhere, let me assure you of one fact: cholesterol is not your enemy. In fact, it is an essential, water-insoluble, body nutrient closely related to vitamin D. The healthy human body produces 2,000 milligrams of cholesterol a day. When you eat foods with more cholesterol, your body slows production. When you eat less cholesterol, your body compensates by producing more. It is transported inside lipoproteins. The two that are prominently referred to are low-density lipoprotein (LDL) and high-density lipoprotein (HDL). Cholesterol transported from the liver by LDL regenerates new cell membranes. Old cholesterol is transported to the liver by HDL to be recycled.

Cholesterol actually plays many roles in good health:

- It holds cell walls together.

- Several hormones, including testosterone and estrogen, are derived from cholesterol.

- Brain cells are made of cholesterol.

- It enables brain synapses to form and fire.

- Psychomotor skills depend on cholesterol.

- It patches damage to arterial walls caused by acid pH.

- It enables cell signaling for guiding and growing nerve axons.

In other words, cholesterol saves lives!

Does high cholesterol exist?

In a word, yes. Just as with sugar or calories, you can overindulge. A diet overly rich in cholesterol may well raise your serum cholesterol level. However, statin drugs do not always succeed in lowering cholesterol, and when they do, they can bring those levels down too much. This can result in:

- Ischemic strokes (80 percent of all strokes are ischemic; 20 percent are hemorrhagic and linked to high cholesterol)[10]

- Behavioral problems and depression due to lowered serotonin, a neurotransmitter in the brain

- Learning disabilities among children

In fact, studies reveal that elderly patients with both low cholesterol and albumin (a blood protein) are 3.5 times more likely to die before those with normal levels.[11]

With organizations such as the American Heart Association; National Heart, Lung, and Blood Institute; and the American College of Cardiology setting ever-lower levels for acceptable cholesterol, these facts are being ignored. Meanwhile, some advocate that anyone with a high (or even moderate) risk of developing high cholesterol be prescribed statins—Lipitor, Crestor, Lescol, Mevacor, and Zocor, to name a few. In some cases they are prescribed for children. On the other side are health practitioners who warn against prescribing statins for anyone. Still, the mainstream buckles under the influence of pharmaceutical companies' dollars. Check with your health care provider before discontinuing any medication.

Achieving balance

Cholesterol is necessary in the right amounts and in proper balance (HDL to LDL). To achieve balance, you must:

1. Feed your body the nutrients it needs to balance itself. For starters, look to the foods you eat. Try to build your diet around whole, organic foods, eaten raw or cooked from scratch. Recent studies confirm that a fiber-rich diet reduces the occurrence of clogged arteries, heart disease, and high cholesterol. General guidelines recommend 20 to 35 grams of fiber per day in the form of fruits, vegetables, beans, and whole grains.

2. Get fit. A regular fitness routine can help balance cholesterol levels.

EAR INFECTIONS: COMMONSENSE CARE

Ear infections are common among children today, and many of them can be linked to a child's diet. Food allergies—especially to milk and dairy products—represent major causes that often get overlooked by pediatricians and family doctors. If your child has frequent ear infections, eliminate dairy products from her diet and see what happens. If they persist, use an elimination diet or pulse testing to see if other foods may be at the root of the problem.

In addition to ear infections, poor nutrition (especially too much sugar in the diet) can lead to colds, flu, and other respiratory illnesses. Sugar compromises the immune system. Did you ever notice how many children get sick after Halloween or the Christmas holidays—when celebrations include even more sugar than they consume the rest of the year? Get your family out of the sugar habit and watch their health improve!

Besides cutting down on sugar, here are some other helpful tips for preventing and treating ear infections in your children:

- Schedule a spinal adjustment to ensure cervical alignment.

- If you suspect allergies are a cause of their problems, be sure they avoid cow's milk, wheat, yeast, eggs, corn, sugar, oranges, and peanut butter.

- Use colloidal silver and garlic to fight infection naturally.

- Build the immune system with a raw-fruit, vegetable, and whole-grain diet.

- Supplement the diet with a high-quality multivitamin/mineral and aloe vera.

- Increase good bacteria in the body by supplementing with L. acidophilus (especially important if antibiotics have been used).

- Feed infants with ear infections in an upright position to help their Eustachian tubes drain.

- Keep them away from cigarette smoke.

- Insert a few drops of warm garlic or olive oil in the ear canal, or use a commercial herbal ear oil with willow bark, olive oil, and garlic.

- Avoid antibiotics, antihistamines, and decongestants. These drugs suppress normal immune response and lead to relapse.

- Increase fluid intake, especially water. Children should drink at least eight glasses of water a day, even when they are not ill.

- Drink 1 to 2 ounces of aloe vera juice with immune-stimulating herbs each day.

ENDOMETRIOSIS:
END IT ONCE AND FOR ALL

A painful condition, endometriosis is caused by an abnormal growth of tissue outside the uterus. Studies have linked endometriosis to the use of popular brand-name menstrual products, such as tampons made from bleached, low-grade cotton or pads containing chemical absorbents.[12] Using a product such as the Diva cup, sea sponge, reusable cloth pads, or organic sanitary products may be your best alternative.

If you suffer from endometriosis, these tips may help.

Nutrition

- Upgrade to a whole foods diet that is based on fresh fruits, vegetables, and whole grains.

- Avoid meat and dairy products, especially those from animals treated with antibiotics or given hormones.

- Supplement your diet with an all-natural, balanced multivitamin/mineral formula that contains absorbable sources of calcium and magnesium.

- Include flaxseed oil in your diet every day. You can use it on salads, stir it into oatmeal, or take one to three 1,000-milligram capsules daily.

- Other helpful supplements include aloe vera juice, garlic, astragalus, pau d'arco, red clover, and alfalfa for vitamin K and iron.

Detoxification

- Detoxifying your body is especially important for women with endometriosis. For starters, drink at least ten glasses of pure, filtered water every day. Include many high-fiber foods in your diet to keep toxins moving through and out of your body.

- Fasting for three days each month before the beginning of your period is beneficial. Fast on steamed, distilled water and freshly juiced fruit and vegetable juices.

- Avoid toxins in your environment, especially dioxins (which can leech from plastic water bottles and dinnerware when frozen or microwaved), dry cleaning fluids, pesticides, and drugs. The chlorine bleaching process used to whiten paper, rayon cotton, and manufactured materials most tampons are made of also can contaminate you with dioxins.

Exercise

Consistent exercise, best started when you are in your early twenties, can decrease estrogen and lessen incidence of endometriosis. However, no matter what your age, it is never too late to start a sensible exercise program.

Remedies

Natural progesterone cream used from ovulation until the first day of your period can help balance estrogen levels.

FLU AND COMMON COLD: COMMONSENSE CARE

Caused by more than two hundred different viruses that attack the upper respiratory tract, the common cold can cause sneezing, watery eyes, runny nose, coughing, and other irritating symptoms. If their immune systems are weak, otherwise healthy adults fight these viruses at least once or twice a year.

When you get a cold and fight it off, it shows your immune system is working. If it takes more than a day or two, your immune system may be compromised. Because children's immune systems are still maturing, they may fight colds off a little more often than adults.

Shorten and win the fight!

- Remain active without overdoing it. The immune system has no pump. Activity moves immune fluids through your body. Walking or light exercise actually helps fight off a cold!

- Double your daily dose of multiple vitamins and minerals. Make sure your multi has adequate vitamin C and zinc.

- Take echinacea at the first sign of symptoms (Echinacea angustifolia is the preferred extract for colds and flu.)

- Increase fluids, especially pure water with lemon. Sip hot liquids; potato peeling broth is great.

- Wash your hands often so you don't spread the virus.

- Avoid over-the-counter remedies, which block normal body functions and hinder immune system activity.

- Do not take antibiotics. They are only effective on specific bacteria, not on viruses that cause cold and flu. Use colloidal silver, garlic, and cayenne pepper as natural alternatives.

Influenza

A highly contagious viral infection spread by coughing and sneezing, influenza infects the upper respiratory tract. When you come down with the flu, you usually experience a dry throat, cough, and body aches. You generally do not feel like doing much of anything, even eating. The flu is more serious in folks over the age of sixty-five.

When you have the flu, you can follow the previously listed recommendations for care of the common cold with one exception—do not remain active. In addition:

- Get plenty of rest.

- Boost your immune system with fresh fruit and vegetable juices.

- Brew and drink peppermint tea to open nasal passages.

- Use cayenne pepper to keep mucus flowing (mucous flow helps eliminate the virus).

- Do not try to lower a fever under 102 degrees. Increased body temperature helps inactivate the virus and speeds up immune system function.

- For a sore throat, gargle, alternating between warm water and hot salt water several times a day (use a quarter teaspoon of salt per 8 ounces of water).

- Cough! Cover your mouth and let it happen. This is your body's way of expelling the virus.

Homemade Healthy Cough Syrup

If coughing interferes with your sleep, use this homemade

cough syrup as an alternative to the toxic, over-the-counter remedies sold by the pharmacy.

½ tsp. slippery elm bark powder
¼ cup honey
½ cup boiling water

Add slippery elm bark powder and honey to boiling water. Stir well. Take 1 teaspoon every three hours.

GOUT AND THE FOODS
THAT SOOTHE IT

Gout, technically known as hyperuricemia, is a painful inflammation caused by uric acid buildup in the joints. It occurs when the liver produces more uric acid than the kidneys can excrete in the urine. Over time, the uric acid crystallizes and settles in the joints, most often the big toe or ankle. This causes swelling, inflammation, stiffness, and pain. Uric acid crystals can damage your nerves, cartilage, and bone.

Gout can be caused by eating too many rich foods or drinking alcohol; it is also a side effect of prescription drugs used to treat high blood pressure, high cholesterol, and digestive upsets. No wonder more than two million people in the United States suffer with gout!

If you have gout, you may have been warned to avoid certain rich foods and alcohol. However, did you know there are also foods that help relieve gout symptoms?

Life is a bowl of cherries

Researchers have found that eating six to eight fresh cherries a day between meals alleviates gout symptoms. If you feel a gout attack coming on, eat twenty to thirty cherries immediately. Cherries help support the health of the connective tissue that is damaged by gout.

They also have an enzyme that neutralizes uric acid and helps prevent inflammation. While you can use frozen and canned cherries, be wary of sugar and additives. A cup of strawberries, a cup of blueberries, or a tablespoon of black cherry juice concentrate with each meal may also help.

Eating generous amounts of any fresh fruits and vegetables can keep uric acid crystals from depositing in the joints. Grapes help your body to eliminate uric acid from your body before it has a chance to crystallize. The potassium in other high-fiber foods can do the same, such as baked potatoes with the skin, yams, spinach, dried peaches or prunes, avocados, cantaloupes, kidney or lima beans, bananas, orange juice, and carrots.

Drink to your health

Although I cautioned earlier to avoid toasting with alcohol, you can make your gout better with the following beverages. Make them a ritual—serve in a cocktail glass, on the rocks, or with a twist of fresh fruit.

- ✓ Water. All of us need to drink six to eight glasses (8 ounces) of water every day. If you have gout, drinking enough water is even more important. Include fresh fruit juices and herbal teas instead of soda pop or caffeinated beverages that drive water and minerals from your body. Keeping your urine diluted helps you to excrete uric acid before crystals have a chance to form.

- ✓ Lemon juice can prevent gout attacks. Drink the juice of one freshly squeezed lemon in a glass of lukewarm water after every meal. It helps your body neutralize the uric acid that triggers gout attacks. (To get more juice out from the lemon, bring it to room temperature and roll it on the counter before squeezing.)

✓ Celery seed tea. As another gout preventative, cook a tablespoon of celery seeds in 2 cups of water till soft. Then strain and drink a half cup, four times a day.

✓ Apple cider vinegar and raw honey. Mix 2 teaspoons of each in a glass of water and drink at mealtime.

A word of caution to dieters

Severe dieting or fasting for extended periods of time can create excess lactic acid. Lactic acid impairs the kidneys so that they cannot excrete uric acid—ouch! More gout pain! Avoid crash diets, which can also drive potassium from your body and increase uric acid formation. If you need to lose weight, follow a sensible diet that includes smaller portions of a variety of healthy, whole foods.

Herbal "wonder food" remedies

The FDA has issued warnings about many common over-the-counter and prescription pain relievers. As I already mentioned, certain foods can help prevent and relieve gout pain. So can some herbal remedies and vitamin/mineral supplements. The following have been commonly used by people with gout. Take these herbs as a tea or extract as directed:

- Alfalfa

- Bilberry

- Black cohosh

- Buchu tea

- Devil's claw

- Garlic

- Hawthorn

- Hydrangea

- Nettle

- Parsley

- Red clover

- Saffron

- Yarrow with nettle

You can use these herbs in a poultice:

- Castor oil. Warm and soak into a piece of flannel and apply to affected area for one hour, twice daily.

- Cayenne pepper. Boil 1 tablespoon in 1 cup of vinegar and 1 cup of water. Dab onto painful joint. Or, mix with wintergreen oil to make a paste and apply.

- Charcoal. Use 1 cup with 3 tablespoons of ground flaxseed and warm water.

- Ginger. Mix ⅓ cup ground ginger into your bath; soak thirty minutes. Rinse well to avoid skin irritation.

- Mullein. Soak leaves in a hot vinegar/water mixture. Pack on the affected area.

- Spearmint. Using leaves, wrap affected area.

- Rose hips. Boil in apple cider vinegar and dab on affected area.

Take these supplements as directed:

- B complex

- Bromelain

- Fish oil capsules

- L-glutamine

- L-glutathione

- L-glycine

- L-methionine

- Magnesium citrate

- Quercetin

- Shark cartilage

- Vitamin C

- Vitamin E

Build good health with good nutrition

Like all health issues, gout will improve as your overall health improves. So maintain a healthy weight and exercise daily. Eat healthy foods—plenty of fresh fruits, vegetables, and whole grains helps control uric acid levels. If possible, consume natural, organic foods, eating them either raw or prepared from scratch. And as your health care provider has probably told you, avoid those foods known to instigate gout flare-ups. Among them are scallops, shrimp, sardines, red meat, gravy, cream sauces, sweets, ice cream, organ meats, turkey, dried peas, legumes, fried foods, caffeine, and alcohol.

Pressure points

Are you still experiencing gout pain? Apply some pressure:

- Press just below the center of your nose toward the upper lip.

- Massage between the ball of your foot and the bottom of your big toe on each foot. On the left foot only, stimulate a point halfway between the base of the little toe and the heel pad.

- Press inward and upward at the base of the skull.

HEARTBURN AND
ACID REFLUX HELP

If you suffer with heartburn, acid reflux, diarrhea, constipation, gas, irritable bowel syndrome (IBS), or other digestive problems, you may be spending a small fortune on over-the-counter or prescription remedies to treat these painful symptoms. The trouble is, symptoms are only a signal—a way your body communicates that something is not right. Taking a Tums or popping a Zelnorm may make you feel better temporarily, but this doesn't address the root cause. Besides masking symptoms—and ignoring what your body is trying to tell you—it can cause health problems to escalate.

Fooling your body never fixes anything

Your digestive system takes charge of a miraculously interactive process that releases and absorbs nutrients from the foods you eat, which are needed for healthy living. In the mouth, enzymes in saliva begin breaking down food. In the stomach, acid and enzymes break down foods and release vitamins, minerals, protein, and fats. Pancreatic juices and bile from the gallbladder get in on the act too. A phenomenal relationship between the brain and gut takes place on a molecular level as neuropeptides and serotonins guide absorption of the released nutrients traveling through the intestines.

Without well-absorbed nutrients, none of the body's systems can enjoy optimum health. When the digestive system is out of balance, it belches, burns, cramps, or explodes. It is important to listen to what your body is trying to tell you—not shut it up with prescription drugs or over-the-counter remedies.

Acid reflux

Acid reflux disease (reflux esophagitis) is a digestive disorder of epidemic proportions. One of every ten Americans suffers from its symptoms. Prilosec, the prescription (also now available in over-the-counter form) used to treat it, is one of the top-selling drugs in the world.

Heartburn and acid reflux occur when gastric (stomach) juices back up into the esophagus. Overeating or eating foods that relax the lower muscles of the esophagus can cause reflux. Other causes include a diet high in junk, fast, and processed foods, and overuse of medications.

Most remedies for acid reflux and heartburn reduce stomach acid. Now, acid isn't always a bad thing. A car battery can't function without acid. Your digestive system can't either. The stomach acid breaks down foods and releases essential nutrients into the body. Furthermore, reducing stomach acid leaves the stomach at the mercy of germs and bacteria that cause food poisoning and other maladies. Laboratory studies with rats have demonstrated that antioxidants from fresh fruits and vegetables can do more to heal acid reflux disease than prescription medications!

These tips might help relieve the discomfort and potentially dangerous disease state that can be caused by acid reflux.

Eating

- Eat smaller amounts of food more often to avoid pressure in the abdomen.

- Avoid such offenders as fried foods, soft drinks, chocolate, coffee, and alcohol.

- Change your diet to include 75 percent raw foods (fruits, vegetables, and whole grains).

- For gentle relief, wash a raw potato and put it in a juicer or blender. Mix with equal parts water and drink as needed.

- At the first sign of trouble, drink a large glass of water.

Body mechanics

- Use gravity to help relieve chronic nighttime heartburn. Do not lie down flat for at least three hours after meals. Elevate the head of your bed with a four-inch block of wood.

- When sleeping, lie on your left side. This keeps the bulk of the stomach lower than its upper opening.

Helpful supplements

- Enhance impaired digestion with live food enzymes.

- Consider taking DGL (deglycyrrhizinised liquorice) or aloe vera to heal the lining of the GI tract.

- Some people find relief from betaine HCL or apple cider vinegar. Use 1 tablespoon before meals for more complete digestion and less delay in emptying the stomach (delay can cause allergic reactions).

- Use natural enzymes for proper digestion. Take before meals. Pancreatin is best.

Avoid the following

- Antacids! An overly acidic stomach does not cause heartburn. Maalox, Rolaids, Mylanta, and other antacids contain aluminum, while Tums and others contain calcium. Both aluminum and calcium can rebound (increase) acidity, causing further discomfort and the need for more antacids. Aluminum is linked to Alzheimer's disease.

- Prescription-strength and over-the-counter medications, such as Pepcid AC, Prilosec, Tagamet, Zantac, and the like. They block normal body processes, impair proper digestion of food, and impede mineral absorption. Long-term use of these medications can damage the stomach lining and increase risk of benign and cancerous tumors.

- Stress and anger.

- Estrogen, e.g. birth control pills and menopause treatments, which can cause the lower muscles of the esophagus to weaken.

- Smoking, which aggravates heartburn.

HIGH BLOOD PRESSURE POINTERS

Blood pressure problems generate a lot of health news today. The only problem is, you may not be aware of whether you have it. The reason: high blood pressure goes about its destructive business in a stealthy manner. You can have it and not even suspect it. So if you haven't had your blood pressure checked recently, get it done immediately. Chances are your county health department, local church, a hospital, or neighborhood medical clinic offers free blood pressure screening. If not, call your doctor's office. You wouldn't take a road trip if you weren't sure about your tire pressure. Your journey to optimal health requires as much attention. Check your blood pressure!

What is high blood pressure?

Blood pressure is the pressure exerted by your blood on the walls of your blood vessels. Blood pressure values are universally stated in millimeters of mercury (mmHg). The systolic pressure is pressure in your arteries during the peak of your cardiac cycle; diastolic pressure measures the pressure at the resting phase of the cardiac cycle.

Nerve impulses cause your arteries to dilate (become larger) or contract (become smaller). When these vessels are wide open, blood flows easily. When they narrow, it is harder for the blood to flow, and the pressure inside them increases. This causes the heart and arteries to work harder and eventually damages them. Other organs, such as the kidney, may become strained too. The higher your blood pressure and the longer it goes untreated, the more you damage your heart, arteries, and kidneys.

What causes high blood pressure?

In approximately 90 percent of high blood pressure cases, doctors can't identify a specific cause. However, high blood pressure is more common in African Americans, middle-age and elderly people, the obese, heavy drinkers, and women taking birth control pills. Some families seem predisposed to high blood pressure, but many with a family history never get it. People with certain chronic diseases—including diabetes, gout, and kidney disease—are more likely to have high blood pressure.

Your blood pressure is determined by four main factors:

1. Your heart rate: how fast your heart pumps.

2. Your blood volume: how much blood you have in your body.

3. The resistance of your blood vessels: the higher the resistance, the higher your blood pressure.

4. Viscosity: the thickness of your blood.

Doctors often warn those with high blood pressure to decrease their salt intake. The reason: sodium may increase blood volume. Doctors also warn people with high cholesterol to lower it, since high cholesterol levels can cause the buildup of plaque in the arteries and increase their resistance. Blood thinners encourage blood to flow more quickly through the vessels.

What does high blood pressure cause?

While most people with high blood pressure don't know what caused it, we do know what high blood pressure causes. It puts you at risk for strokes, heart attacks, heart failure, arterial aneurysms, and is the second leading cause of kidney failure in people with diabetes.

Take the pressure off

Making lifestyle changes can help you keep your blood pressure at healthy levels. Try these:

- Reduce the amount of fatty foods you eat. Eliminate saturated fats, which are the worst culprits! All animal fats—those found in meat, poultry, and dairy products—are saturated. Processed and fast foods also have saturated fats. Even vegetable oils can be saturated; for example, palm, palm kernel, and coconut oils are saturated fats. All vegetable oils become saturated when they undergo a food processing technique called hydrogenation. Read the label—if the product contains hydrogenated vegetable oil, it contains unhealthy, saturated fats.

- Quit smoking and drink less (or no) alcohol. Both can contribute to high blood pressure as well as heart attack and stroke.

- Build your diet around whole, organic foods, eaten raw or cooked from scratch. Recent studies confirm that a fiber-rich diet reduces the occurrence of clogged arteries—which means lower blood pressure. You will find fiber in fresh fruits, vegetables, legumes (beans), and whole grains.

Perhaps you believe it would be easier to just take medications to control high blood pressure. You likely know some people who do. While medications do have their time and place, they also have side effects. If you can maintain healthy blood pressure without drugs, you won't have to worry about these potentially dangerous side effects.

Drug dangers

Watch out for these problems with various substances.

- **Diuretics (water pills).** These reduce blood volume by removing excess salt and water from the body. Generic label, with corresponding brands in parentheses: hydrochlorothiazide (Carozide, Diaqua, Esidrix, HydroDIURIL, Microzide, and Oretic). Known side effects include dizziness, lack of urination, muscle weakness and cramping, irregular heartbeat.

- **Vasodilators.** These improve blood flow by relaxing muscles in blood vessel walls to open them up. Generic and corresponding brands: guanabenz (Wytensin), dozazosin (Carduara), guanfacine (Tenex), guanethidine (Ismelin), methyldopa (Aldomet), prazosin (Minipress), terazosin (Hytrin), reserpine (Diupres), hydralazine (Apresoline), minoxidil (Loniten). Known side effects are rapid heartbeat, headache, fluid retention, impotence, gastrointestinal problems (hydralazine), and hair growth (monoxidil).

- **Alpha blockers.** These improve blood flow by reducing nerve impulses to blood vessel muscles. Generic and corresponding brands: doxazosin (Cardura), clonidine (Catapres), prazosin (Minipress), guanfacine (Tenex).

Known side effects include rapid heartbeat, headache, fluid retention, impotence, gastrointestinal problems, nightmares, numbness or tingling in the hands, and nausea.

IBS: A PERSONAL AND SOCIAL NIGHTMARE

Irritable bowel syndrome (IBS) is a combination of symptoms that lead to tenderness, throbbing and agonizing pain, accompanied by bloating, embarrassing flatulence, and either incontinent diarrhea or obstructive constipation. Other symptoms include:

- Acid reflux

- Groin pain and contractions

- Stomach cramping and pain

- Exhaustion

- Lower back pain

- Shooting pain in your hips and legs

- Inability to mentally focus

- Anxiety attacks

- Changes in heart rate and light-headedness

- Constant weight gain

These symptoms arise when your digestion system fails to completely digest your food. Eighty percent of IBS patients report it as a progressive condition that—from the point of experiencing the first symptom—can disable them within only a few years

Over the past decade IBS has become the most widespread digestive ailment in the United States. Traditional medicine has no diagnosis for it, so it gets labeled as a syndrome. Most physicians do not know how to remedy IBS; too often medical treatments are inadequate and ineffective.

If you suffer from IBS or other digestive upsets, you may be spending a lot of money on over-the-counter and prescription remedies to treat painful symptoms. The trouble is, symptoms are only a signal—a way your body communicates that something is not right. As I said earlier in the section on stomach trouble, taking a Tums or popping a Zelnorm may help temporarily but ignore the root cause. This can cause problems to get worse.

Often, prescribed antispasmodic drugs (such as Lomotil) and diarrhea remedies (Imodium A-D) slow intestinal functions, which can cause serious side effects and dependency. Steroid drugs, cholesterol-lowering drugs, and sulfasalazines (such as Azulfidine, prescribed for ulcerative colitis) can make matters worse as they can interfere with absorption in the intestines. Addictive tranquilizers and antidepressants can be equally dangerous.

IBS: the cause

Many have speculated on the causes of IBS: genetics, infection, immune disorders, stress, and diet. IBS is much more common in societies with a Western diet, such as that eaten in the United States. Not surprisingly, IBS virtually does not exist in societies where people eat their food fresh and prepare it from scratch, without additives or preservatives. Keeping that in mind, the first way to attack IBS is to defend your digestive system from the foods that are upsetting it. So if you experience the symptoms of IBS, start by avoiding sugar, caffeine, alcohol, fatty foods, carbonated beverages, and processed foods.

Food allergies can also trigger IBS symptoms. Common triggers are cow's milk, wheat, yeast, eggs, soy, corn, chocolate, and citrus fruits.

Prescription medicines, lack of sleep, and stress can also lead to IBS.

Finding relief

Because a poor diet causes IBS, a good diet can help heal it. Eat healthy foods; a diet that includes plenty of fresh fruits, vegetables, and whole grains is easier to digest. Consume natural, organic foods, either raw or prepared from scratch. Live, uncooked food is better when possible.

Meat and dairy products may contribute to digestive upsets. Eat slowly, while you're relaxed, and chew every bite well. Digestion starts in the mouth—your saliva has enzymes that start the process! Remember too that processed, fast, and refined foods contain large amounts of fat, sugar, and irritating additives. The time you save in the fast-food line may be wasted later when you are sidelined by pain and extra time in the bathroom.

To decrease inflammation, take a tablespoon of flaxseed oil every day. You can use this as a salad dressing or stir it into hot cereals or juice. Aloe vera can help heal irritated intestinal walls. A good multi-vitamin/mineral supplement can help your body recover from months of poor food absorption. To rebalance your digestive system, include a fiber supplement, acidophilus, and a good enzyme formula.

Since stress is also a factor contributing to IBS, manage it with exercise, relaxation, and plenty of sleep. Schedule a therapeutic massage, take a walk outdoors every day, or wind down at night with a nice hot soak in the tub.

INSULIN RESISTANCE, DIABETES, AND SYNDROME X

The Obesity Association states that 127 million (64.5 percent) of US adults are overweight, and 60 million (30.5 percent) are obese.[13] Diabetes among Americans is close to a pandemic. Heart disease, with help from its cohorts—high blood pressure and high cholesterol—is the nation's number one killer.[14] Studies have found a common denominator among all of these conditions: insulin resistance.[15]

What is insulin resistance?

A hormone secreted by the pancreas, insulin unlocks cells so they can convert glucose into energy. When insulin resistance occurs, the cells stay locked tight and glucose builds up in the blood, which causes high blood sugar. As a result, the pancreas manufactures more insulin. The excess insulin in the blood causes the liver to manufacture excess cholesterol.

In severe cases of insulin resistance, the cells fail to unlock, no matter how much insulin the pancreas secretes. Over time, the pancreas' ability to release insulin declines and blood sugar levels rise. The ultimate result? Type 2 diabetes. However, before people even suspect insulin resistance, they may find maintaining a healthy weight is difficult or impossible.

Signs of insulin resistance

- Excess fat around the waist and buttocks

- Inability to lose weight and maintain weight loss

- Lack of energy, especially in the afternoon and after meals

- Lack of concentration and mental fatigue

Fueling weight gain, foiling weight loss

During digestion, the body turns carbohydrates—bread, pasta, rice, and sweets—into glucose (sugar). The standard American diet includes many highly processed carbohydrates and refined sugars, which means the pancreas must work overtime to manufacture enough insulin to handle all this glucose. When the cells say "enough is enough" and become insulin-resistant, the body stores excess blood sugar as fat. When cells develop insulin resistance, the body goes into hibernation mode, making diabetics tired and always hungry.

Insulin resistance causes the body to store more fat while preventing the body from burning fat as energy (decreased metabolism). Insulin resistance is more than a trait found in overweight and obese people—it may well be the root cause of their weight problem. In fact, people following popular, low-fat diets may encounter an additional challenge to weight loss.

Syndrome X: the disease link

The link of insulin resistance with life-threatening diseases has turned it into a billion-dollar watchword in medical circles. Syndrome X is the term used for a cluster of risk factors for heart disease: hypertriglyceridemia (high blood lipids), low HDL-cholesterol, hyperinsulinemia (high blood insulin), hyperglycemia (high blood glucose), and hypertension (high blood pressure). All these risk factors have been linked to insulin resistance.

Of the 60 million Americans diagnosed with insulin resistance, one in four will develop type 2 diabetes.[16] Insulin resistance also increases risk of stroke and blood lipid imbalances that lead to atherosclerosis (hardening of the arteries). The excess insulin in the blood triggers the liver to manufacture more cholesterol.

A diagnosis of insulin resistance is usually not made until people are diagnosed with one of the above diseases. Insulin resistance can be treated with two prescription drugs: pioglitazone and glimepirid. As with many pharmaceuticals, their use can result in a barrage of side effects, including weight gain.

Reversing insulin resistance

Reversing insulin resistance starts with practical advice. Be active, exercise on a regular basis, count calories, and eat well—preferably a daily diet that includes:

- Five to nine servings of fruits and vegetables (the fresher the better)

- Five to 8 ounces of protein

- Two to five servings of 100 percent whole grains (bread, pasta, rice)

- Two to three servings of calcium rich foods.

- Two to 3 tablespoons of healthy fats

- A good, daily multiple vitamin containing chromium and vanadium, two vital blood-sugar regulators

As I have said throughout this book, organic foods are always preferable, as is cooking from scratch. Additives used in processed foods, such as high-fructose corn syrup, lead to hard-to-lose belly fat. Be sensible about good eating too. Don't waste your time on fad diets or just wait for a diagnosis of disease. Work with your body naturally by eating right and getting adequate physical activity.

MENOPAUSE AND NATIVE AMERICAN HERBAL REMEDIES

Long before Europeans colonized the Americas, Native Americans were wisely using the root of black cohosh to treat menstrual difficulties, ease menopausal symptoms, and aid childbirth. The Delaware tribe combined black cohosh with other herbs as a tonic for female members. The Iroquois brewed a strong tea from the root and also used it as a footbath and to treat rheumatism. Likewise, the Cherokee used the roots to treat many different female conditions.

American herbalists learned about the efficacy of black cohosh from their Native American neighbors. Its importance as a medicinal herb was first recorded in 1801. From 1820 to 1926, black cohosh root was listed as an official drug by the United States Pharmacopoeia, the organization that sets standards for all prescriptions, over-the-counter medications, and other health care products sold in the country. Throughout the 1800s white physicians routinely prescribed it to their patients. Black cohosh sometimes carried different names, such as black snakeroot and macrotys. Today black cohosh goes by the scientific names *Actaea racemosa* and *Cimicifuga racemosa* and is also referred to as black baneberry.

An herbal renaissance

It has taken centuries for mainstream America to recognize the wisdom and beauty found in the beliefs and practices of our Native American neighbors. Many of us have come to respect their stewardship of the land and reverence for animal life. We are also learning the efficacy of their healing practices, including the use of herbs.

The physician that introduced echinacea to the white medical community in the mid-1800s, Dr. John King, told his obstetrics students that black cohosh was his favorite remedy. He used it in his practice, making it his primary treatment for any abnormalities in females' principal reproductive organs. King's work piqued the attention of the medical community in Germany, where black cohosh still remains a commonly prescribed remedy.

In modern times the American medical community has looked to Germany for documented experience with this useful traditional American Indian remedy. Black cohosh has remained a popular remedy for menopausal symptoms there for the past 150 years.

By 1962 more than a dozen clinical studies involving more than fifteen hundred participants had been published on the use of black cohosh in the treatment of premenopausal and menopausal symptoms. It was proven to reduce the severity and duration of hot flashes, relieve night sweats, and improve depressive moods. Studies in the 1980s and 1990s not only confirmed these conclusions but also showed black cohosh to be a safe, effective alternative to estrogen replacement therapy—which puts women at substantial risk for many deadly and dangerous side effects.

What causes menopausal symptoms?

Declining estrogen levels are at the heart of menopausal symptoms. However, today's lifestyles can make them worse. Not only do our diets often consist of highly processed foods, but we also breathe polluted air and drink fluoridated or chlorinated water. Then there are our harried schedules and information overload, which drives up stress levels. Add in the fact that many of us fail to take time to enjoy exercise, fresh air, and sunshine, and we become walking time bombs.

Consider menopausal links to physical problems:

- What causes hot flashes? Instability in your small blood arteries and capillaries leads them to dilate.

- What causes the blues? Estrogens are psychoactive hormones; their changing levels may cause you to feel depressed, anxious, or experience mood swings. You may feel a profound sense of loss as you lose your fertility.

- What causes vaginal dryness and loss of libido? Less estrogen can mean lower libido. When your body ceases to create natural lubrication, sex may be uncomfortable or even painful. As estrogen decreases, your skin may become drier and bruise easily.

- You may have problems with incontinence. Don't be alarmed. The following diet suggestions, along with an herbal supplement that includes black cohosh, can help see you through.

1. First, include plant estrogens in your diet: organic soy products and tofu, linseeds, chickpeas, lentils, and mung beans.

2. Next, reduce your sugar and junk foods.

3. Monitor your salt intake; pay attention to sodium levels on nutrition labels and aim for those with low (or no) content. Avoid spicy food, hot drinks, and alcohol, which can aggravate hot flashes.

4. Limit red meat to one or two portions each week.

5. Use safflower, sunflower, olive, sesame, and rapeseed oils instead of animal fats.

6. Include foods high in calcium and magnesium: milk, leafy green vegetables, unsalted nuts and seeds, whole grains, and sardines.

7. Consume natural, organic foods: raw or prepared from scratch. Include fresh fruits, vegetables, and whole grains.

8. Drink eight to twelve glasses of pure water daily.

OSTEOPOROSIS: NO BONES ABOUT IT!

A progressive disorder, osteoporosis causes your bones to become weaker and weaker, leading to changes in posture and putting you at risk for bone fractures and life-changing complications. If you have noticed a gradual loss of height, your shoulders have become more rounded, or you have general aches and pains throughout your body, you may be a victim of osteoporosis.

Preventing and controlling osteoporosis calls for a three-prong attack: exercise, nutrition, and sunshine.

Exercise

Consistent, moderate, weight-bearing exercise not only decreases bone loss, but it also increases bone mass. When you are inactive, calcium—the bone-building mineral—leeches out of your system in urine and stools. The following forms of exercise will benefit people at risk of osteoporosis or who have already received that diagnosis.

Strength training. Free weights, weight machines, resistance bands, or water exercises strengthen the muscles and bones in your arms and upper spine. They also slow mineral loss from bones and maintain flexibility in the spine.

Weight-bearing aerobic exercise. Walking, dancing, low-impact aerobics, and gardening work directly on the bones in legs, hips, and lower spine to slow mineral loss. They also reduce the risk of heart disease.

Flexibility exercises. Increasing joint mobility improves posture. Chest and shoulder stretches may be helpful, as may prone push-ups. Perform stretches after your muscles are warmed up and at the end of your exercise session.

Movements to avoid if you have osteoporosis include high-impact exercises, such as jumping, running, or jogging. These can lead to fractures in weakened bones. Also avoid exercises in which you bend forward and twist your waist, such as touching your toes, doing sit-ups, or using a rowing machine. These compress the bones in your spine. Other activities you should avoid because they require these actions are golf, tennis, bowling, and some yoga poses.

Nutrition

Calcium deficiency and bone loss are often symptoms of a larger dietary problem. Good sources of calcium include broccoli, dark leafy greens, kelp, oats, sesame seeds, soybeans, and wheat germ. In addition, eat a whole foods diet based on fresh fruits, vegetables, and 100 percent whole grains. Be sure to include fresh garlic and onions as you cook healthy dinners from scratch. Both contain sulfur, another mineral important for strong bones. Organic soy products can also slow bone loss. (Beware—soybeans that are not certified organic may be genetically modified and dangerous for your overall health.)

Take a high quality, natural multivitamin/mineral formula that contains the vitamins C, D, E, K, B_6, and B_{12} and the minerals calcium, magnesium, boron, zinc, copper, silicon, manganese, and chromium. Chromium improves bone density and insulin efficiency. Avoid synthetic vitamins and poorly vitalized forms of calcium, such as calcium carbonate.

Instead of exposing yourself to the risks of prescription bone-loss drugs or dangerous hormone replacement therapy, supplement with DHEA, a natural alternative to hormone replacement.

Calcium hazards to avoid:

- Excess protein, especially from meat and dairy products.

- Sugar. Sugar promotes calcium loss. So do coffee (caffeine), alcohol, and smoking.

- Carbonated beverages (soda pop). These contain phosphates, which leech calcium and other bone-friendly minerals from your system into your urine.

A final step

Last but not least, get out in the fresh air and enjoy the sunshine whenever you can. Exposure to sunlight, even just fifteen minutes on the face, arms and hands, helps your body build bones with stored calcium.

PULSE TESTING FOR FOOD ALLERGIES

The pulse test is a good way to identify foods that cause allergic reactions, but you should only test one food a day. Here's how:

- Before getting out of bed in the morning, take your resting pulse. Using your index finger on the thumb side of your other wrist, count the number of beats you feel in one minute. Write this number down.

- Next, eat the food you want to test. Only eat one food or you won't know which caused the reaction.

- Remain in a resting position. After ten minutes, take your pulse again. Record this number.

- Remain in a resting position. After an additional ten minutes, take your pulse again. Record this number.

- Compare your original pulse rate with the next two readings. If you experienced an increase of ten or more beats per minute, chances are you have identified a food that causes you to have an allergic reaction. Eliminate this food from your diet.

SINUS PROBLEMS: A REAL DRAIN!

An inflammation of the mucous membranes in the nasal sinuses, sinusitis can be caused by food allergies, infection, or other factors that weaken the immune system. Symptoms include facial pain or tenderness, headaches, earaches, toothaches, low-grade fevers, or difficulty breathing through your nose. When you have a sinus problem, keep these two goals in mind:

1. Preventing the sinus membranes from further swelling

2. Assisting the body in draining the mucus.

To accomplish these goals, follow these suggestions:

Prevent swelling

- Identify foods that cause allergies and eliminate them from your diet. The most common culprits are milk, wheat, yeast, eggs, corn, citrus fruits, and peanut butter. To identify which foods cause you problems, use an elimination diet or the pulse testing I reviewed in the last section.

- Eat a 75 percent raw diet consisting of fruits, vegetables, and whole grains.

- Upgrade your nutrition with a high-quality multivitamin/mineral formula that includes plenty of antioxidants, vitamins A, C, and E, and selenium.

- Eliminate sugar (do not substitute artificial sweeteners; although a moderate amount of stevia may be tolerated).

Promote drainage

- Breathe steam under a towel tent for ten minutes at a time, several times a day. You can add eucalyptus or menthol to increase effectiveness.

- Apply a warm towel to your sinus area for twenty minutes. Then, lie down with your head lower than the rest of your body to help your sinuses drain.

- Irrigate your sinuses with a mixture of 1 cup of warm water, a half teaspoon of salt, and a pinch of baking soda. Syringe into your nostrils and gently blow your nose.

- Use the herb Ma Huang to relieve congestion and swelling. In difficult cases, use goldenseal, a natural anti-infective and immune stimulator, and bromelain to help break up the mucus.

- Replace healthy bacterial flora with L. acidophilus.

Avoid antibiotics, antihistamines, and nose sprays

If you suspect infection, use colloidal silver, garlic, pycnogenols, and aloe vera juice to boost your immune system. Antihistamines and nose sprays interfere with normal sinus drainage.

THYROID HEALTH: COMMONSENSE TIPS

When your thyroid is not functioning at full speed, your whole health suffers. Thyroid problems are frequently related to food allergies. So your first step is to identify offending foods through an elimination diet or pulse testing. (See Pulse Testing for Food Allergies.)

Next, rule out any other contributing factors, such as heavy metal poisoning, parasites, hypoglycemia, and yeast syndrome. These can all impact thyroid health.

Use a proper diet

- Eat four to five smaller meals every day.

- Drink eight to twelve glasses of pure, filtered water daily.

- Begin with a 50 percent raw food diet, based on fruits, vegetables, and 100 percent whole grains.

- Eat a variety of whole grains; include millet and brown rice.

- For protein, eat raw nuts, seeds, and cold-water fish (e.g., salmon).

- Sprout your own lentils or alfalfa seeds, or purchase fresh organic sprouts to add to salads and sandwiches.

- Avoid animal products (i.e., meat and dairy).

- Avoid nightshade vegetables: potatoes, tomatoes, peppers, eggplant, and tobacco.

- Abstain from sugar, coffee (caffeine), and alcohol.

- Supplement your diet with a high-quality multivitamin and mineral formula that includes natural antioxidants and glandulars (adrenal and liver).

- Supplement with chlorophyll tablet or "green" drinks.

Daily habits

- Establish a consistent exercise routine that includes stretching and light to moderate exercise.

- Sleep at least eight hours every night.

- Cleanse your colon with psyllium or cascara sagrada herbs.

- Alternate hot and cold showers to stimulate blood circulation.

WHAT HAPPENS WHEN I DRINK CERTAIN BEVERAGES?

You have likely heard the old cliché "You are what you eat." Well, you are what you drink too. Only during the past few decades did soda pop and sugary juice drinks become dietary staples, served with almost every meal. If that weren't bad enough, today most milk sold in grocery stores is laced with hormones and antibiotics. While millions depend on coffee to get started in the morning or alcohol to unwind, have they really considered what dependence on these substances is doing to their health? This is why the best beverage is the no-calorie, no-sodium, healthy, God-given liquid: pure water.

What about soft drinks?

Don't be fooled by their name—soft drinks are hard on your body. They are manufactured with excess sugar and phosphates; both cause calcium loss in urine. Excess dietary sugar also turns into fat and depletes the body of B vitamins, especially B_1 (thiamin). Low B_1 can cause mood changes and behavior disorders. Sugar also directly suppresses the immune system by lowering white blood cell activity.

In addition, soft drinks lower your pH level, acidifying the body and promoting aging and free radical damage. It takes more than thirty-two glasses of pure water to undo the affects of one soft drink.

What about diet soft drinks?

They are just as dangerous as their fructrose-sweetened cousin. NutraSweet, Splenda, and other artificial sweeteners are highly toxic. NutraSweet (aspartame) breaks down in the body into poisonous methanol and cancer-causing formaldehyde. Diet products containing NutraSweet can cause dozens of symptoms, including headache, fatigue, irritability, depression, seizures, an unnatural craving for sweets, and more. Forget about losing any extra pounds; this artificial sweetener causes weight gain.

What about cow's milk?

If you are a baby cow, milk is the drink for you. Otherwise, it is a source of problems. Milk causes calcium loss in urine, provokes allergies, and can cause any number of negative symptoms. Dairy farmers routinely feed their cows hormones and antibiotics. Growth hormones in milk can promote tumor growth and early puberty; the latter can destroy good bacteria in your GI track. Milk can also contain parasites. If you must drink milk, buy organic. Organic rice or soy milk makes a great substitute.

You might ask, "Don't kids need cow's milk?" As a doctor and father of four children, I recommend that you give your kids organic rice milk or soy milk. Keep in mind that God designed cows' milk for *calves*. It is astonishingly high in protein and fat. Though advertised as a great source of calcium, it causes calcium depletion. Cows' milk's high protein content causes the kidneys to lose calcium in the urine. So even though it contains a large amount of calcium, drinking it results in a net *loss* of calcium.

Cows' milk also provokes allergies (starting with lactose intolerance). When homogenized in processing, then it gets really scary. Homogenization and pasteurization turn milk into a man-made food containing more health liabilities than assets. Cow's milk is best left to baby cows.

What about coffee?

Although caffeine gives you a morning "kick," it also kicks your kidneys into distress. Do you have chronic back pain? Knee pain? Try cutting out caffeine and see what happens. Coffee also causes excess loss of calcium in the urine and creates the potential for cadmium toxicity. Cadmium replaces the body's zinc stores, a health issue since zinc is one of the most important minerals for a strong immune system and proper T-cells. Cadmium also promotes cancerous changes in the cells of the body.

In addition, don't think that decaffeinated coffee is an acceptable alternative. It still contains the cadmium and other chemicals used in processing, which make it even more toxic.

Instead of either kind of coffee, try safer, natural alternatives for energy and clearer, more focused thinking. Among these are ginkgo biloba, yerba mate tea, and ginseng.

What about alcohol?

It may be popular for relaxation, but alcohol is a poison that directly damages the brain, liver, pancreas, and small intestine. The danger of killing brain cells is obvious. In the liver, fatty accumulations can lead to hepatitis, cirrhosis, and eventually death. Damage to the pancreas can lead to diabetes.

Effects on the small intestine lead to poor absorption of all nutrients, especially the fat-soluble vitamins (A, D, E, and K), the B vitamins, folic acid, and vitamin C. This is particularly disturbing because many of these protect the body from free-radical damage, which promotes aging and diseases associated with aging (including heart disease, cancer, and arthritis). Alcohol can increase free-radical formation, making it a double-edged sword that speeds aging. It also suppresses the immune system and depletes the body of zinc (a major immune-stimulating mineral).

Leading alcohol-related causes of death

1. Car accidents

2. Cirrhosis of the liver

3. Pneumonia

4. Suicide

5. Murder

Get wet!

According to the biblical story of Creation, on the first day God created water. Water is the basis for life on earth and the life of your body. The healthy adult body is 65 percent water, while the healthy brain consists of between 75 and 80 percent water. It is easy to see why water should be your beverage of choice. For optimum health, drink at least eight 8-ounce glasses of pure, filtered, or distilled water every day. Municipal water supplies add chemicals, such as fluoride, which has been linked to bone cancer, and chlorine, which kills beneficial intestinal flora, is linked to cancers, and can impair skin, hair, and nail health.

Part of the mystique of the other beverages I warned about is the rituals that go with them. Turn water into its own celebration. Drink yours in a stemmed glass, on ice, or hot (brewed as an herbal tea) in your favorite mug. You can relax, chat, play board games, and celebrate with water as easily as more harmful substances. So enjoy, give thanks, and be healthy!

YEAST INFECTIONS: A CLEAR AND PRESENT DANGER

Yeast (*Candida albicans*) naturally lives in a healthy digestive system— the mouth, throat, intestines, and genitourinary tract. It is a normal bowel flora that destroys harmful bacteria. However, when Candida overgrows, it shifts into a fungal form that invades the body. It then causes vaginal yeast infections, oral thrush infestations, and—when the fungal rhizoids penetrate intestinal walls—leaky gut syndrome. The latter is a condition that allows toxins, undigested food, bacteria, and yeast to enter the bloodstream.

Symptoms of Candida fungal infection

- Cravings for sweets

- Overall feeling of poor health

- Embarrassing rectal or vaginal itch

- Splotchy skin or rashes

If your body has indeed been overrun by *Candida albicans*, you may also experience:

- Lack of energy: sleepiness, fatigue, and feelings of tiredness and/or insomnia

- Pain: muscle aches, headache, painful joints, or numbness

- Mental fog: inability to focus, mood swings, depression, crying jags, and irritability

- Sinus pain, dizziness, and sore throat

- Bad breath and body odor

- Gastrointestinal problems: constipation, diarrhea, bloating, gas, irritable bowel syndrome, abdominal cramps

- Respiratory problems: coughing, wheezing, or shortness of breath

- Loss of libido

If you have any of the following medical conditions, you may also be a victim of Candida fungal infection:

- PMS and menstrual irregularities

- Fibromyalgia and chronic fatigue syndrome

- Sexual dysfunction

- Asthma and allergies

- Food allergies

- Ear infections

- Psoriasis and athlete's foot

- Urinary tract problems

- Multiple sclerosis

- Migraines

Common signs of Candida overgrowth

When you hear the term *yeast infection*, two well-known manifestations of this condition may come to mind.

Oral thrush

A yeast infection on your tongue and inside your cheeks, oral thrush results in creamy white lesions that may bleed slightly when you scrape them or brush your teeth. If left untreated, thrush can spread to the roof of your mouth, gums, tonsils, and the back of your throat. Thrush occurs more often in babies, toddlers, older adults, and those with compromised immune systems. Severe thrush can travel down the esophagus and into the stomach, causing painful swallowing or the sensation that something is stuck in your throat.

Home remedies include eating plain yogurt or applying a solution made of 1 teaspoon of baking soda or 1 tablespoon of vinegar dissolved in 8 ounces of water. You can also break open a capsule of acidophilus and rub it on the lesions.

Vaginal yeast infections

If you watch TV, surf the Internet, or read a magazine, you have likely encountered commercials or advertisements promoting various products to eliminate these infections. A vaginal yeast infection results in a thick, white, cottage-cheese-like discharge that causes painful irritation, constant itching, and pain during intercourse. Home remedies include using plain, unsweetened yogurt or a peeled garlic clove wrapped in gauze as suppositories. When using these, dress so as not to restrict airflow. Wear a skirt or loose-fitting pants, no panties to bed, and avoid tight jeans and pantyhose.

If you find that thrush or vaginal yeast infections are a recurrent occurrence, most likely the yeast overgrowth is not limited to these areas of inflammation.

The yeast epidemic

Many modern health care and hygiene practices stimulate Candida fungal infection. One common culprit is antibiotics. The problem with them is that, along with the harmful bacteria in our bodies, antibiotics kill the good bacteria. These good bacteria balance naturally occurring Candida, so when they are eliminated from the body, Candida overgrows. Chemicals, chlorinated water, antibiotics used in farm animals and meat processing, and pesticides in the environment stimulate Candida overgrowth. Our sugary foods feed Candida and cause overgrowth, as well. Virtually everyone today is at risk for Candida fungal infection.

Other factors that raise the risk of Candida overgrowth include:

- Steroids

- Uncontrolled diabetes

- Hormonal changes: pregnancy, using birth control pills, and menopause

Bubble baths, vaginal contraceptives, damp or tight-fitting clothing, and feminine hygiene sprays and deodorants can also increase susceptibility to yeast infections.

Are you at risk for Candida overgrowth?

If you respond yes to seven or more of the following questions, you probably have a Candida overgrowth issue.

1. Has your doctor routinely prescribed antibiotics for ear infections, acne, respiratory infections, or other reasons?

2. Have you ever been on a course of prednisone, steroids, or birth control pills?

3. Do you eat a lot of dairy products, poultry, beef, or pork from animals raised on antibiotics?

4. Do you feel sick all over but your doctor doesn't know why?

5. Is it sometimes hard to stay focused because you feel "spacey"?

6. Do cigarette smoke, perfumes, or home fragrances give you headaches?

7. Do you have irritable bowel syndrome or any of its symptoms: constipation, diarrhea, bloating, excess gas?

8. Do you crave sugar?

9. Do you suffer with PMS, menstrual irregularities, low libido, or sexual dysfunction?

10. Do you routinely suffer with vaginitis, rectal itch, or thrush?

11. Do you have light "splotches" on the skin of your arms or legs, or have dry skin or easily irritated skin?

Dangers of Candida overgrowth

When Candida transforms from yeast into dangerous fungi, it seeps toxins that block normal nutrient absorption. Candida rhizoids take deep root in your intestinal walls, causing symptoms of irritable bowel syndrome. Eventually rhizoids perforate the intestines, causing leaky gut syndrome. When Candida toxins get into your bloodstream, systemic Candida can invade all of your organs and tissues.

Untreated Candida can trigger bowel disorders, food intolerance, environmental sensitivities, allergies, and asthma. Candida can set off autoimmune disorders, such as chronic fatigue syndrome and fibromyalgia, where your body begins attacking itself at the cellular level.

Overcoming Candida overgrowth

Cut out sugar

Yeast is an organism. Like all living creatures, it needs food to live and multiply. What feeds yeast? Sugar. Have you ever baked homemade bread? If so, you may observed what happens when you mix the baking yeast with warm liquid and sugar in a bowl—it grows, froths, and, when mixed with the other ingredients, its continued growth causes the bread to expand and rise.

The average American eats 53 teaspoons of sugar a day. If you are serious about stopping Candida overgrowth in its tracks, cut sugar out of your diet. This doesn't only mean sugary soft drinks, cookies, candy, and sweets. Sugar hides in most of today's processed foods. Read the labels and root out sugar and all its forms—such as high-fructose corn syrup—from your diet. You will starve the yeast and enjoy other health benefits as well.

Eat healthy foods

Focus on God-made foods: fresh fruits and vegetables, nuts and seeds, unprocessed oils, and limited quantities of antibiotic-free meat, fish, and eggs. Drink eight to twelve glasses of pure, filtered water every day. Avoid flavored waters. If they don't contain sugar, they do contain artificial sweeteners that can wreak even more havoc on your health. If desired, substitute unsweetened green tea for up to four daily water servings.

Also, eating organic, plain yogurt with active probiotic cultures can help reintroduce balance to your system.

Rule out food triggers

To rule out food allergy culprits in your diet, avoid the following foods for two weeks. Then introduce them, one at a time, to see what ill effects they may have on you:

- Yeast (breads made with it)

- Food coloring and additives

- Milk and dairy products

- Processed and packaged foods

- Wheat, oats, and rice

- Beef, pork, chicken, and eggs

- Coffee, tea, and fruit punch

- Citrus fruits, corn, tomatoes, and white potatoes

- Chocolate

Supplement your diet

Choose a high-quality brand of supplement as recommended by your physician, alternative health care practitioner, or trusted nutraceutical source.

- Probiotics, such as acidophilus, are the friendly bacteria that the Candida has overrun. These helpful microorganisms help maintain the health of your digestive tract.

- Digestive enzymes can help maintain a natural, healthy digestion and reduce the occurrence of Candida in the intestines.

- Herbals that help inhibit the growth of Candida include usnea, Spilanthes, pau d'arco, oregano oil, black walnut, grapefruit seed extract, garlic, beta carotene, and biotin.

- Daily multivitamin and mineral supplements help your body fight off Candida overgrowth.

NOTES

INTRODUCTION:
GOD WANTS YOU TO ENROLL IN HIS PERFECT HEALTH PLAN

1. The Quotations Page, http://www.quotationspage.com/quote/38576
.html (accessed October 26, 2011).

CHAPTER 1
KEY 1: LEARN TO RELAX LIKE THE LORD

1. The Quotations Page, http://www.quotationspage.com/quote/38977
.html (accessed January 17, 2012).

2. Helpguide, "Laughter Is the Best Medicine: The Health Benefits
of Humor and Laughter," http://www.helpguide.org/life/humor_
laughter_health.htm (accessed October 24, 2011).

3. "University of Maryland School of Medicine Shows Laughter Helps
Blood Vessels Function Better," http://www.umm.edu/news/releases/
laughter2.htm (accessed October 24, 2011).

CHAPTER 2
KEY 2: GET TO BED ON TIME: SLEEP AND THE GREAT HEALER

1. John Berman and Enjoli Francis, "AAA Says 2-of-5 Drivers Admit
Nodding Off at the Wheel," ABC News, November 8, 2010, http://
abcnews.go.com/WN/driving-sleepy-common-deadly-thought-aaa
-research-finds/story?id=12088552 (accessed January 17, 2012).

2. Scanlan Law Group, "Fatal Crash Caused by Sleeping Truck Driver
Yields $1.2 Million for Victims," http://www.scanlanlawgroup.com/
lawyer-attorney-1159215.html (accessed January 17, 2012).

3. KSDK.com, "Four Killed in Virginia Bus Rollover Crash,"
Associated Press, May 31, 2011, http://www.ksdk.com/news/
article/261045/3/Virginia-bus-crash-claims-four-lives (accessed
January 17, 2012).

4. Coastal Coast News, "Sleepy Driver Causes Major Injury Crash
on Highway 1," http://www.kionrightnow.com/story/14991378/
accident-in-santa-cruz-closes-down-part-of-highway-1 (accessed
January 17, 2012).

5. News Channel 7, "Coroner: I-85 Collision Caused by Tractor Trailer Truck Driver Asleep at Wheel," August 1, 2011, http://www2.wspa .com/news/2011/jul/30/14/i-85-north-bound-anderson-county-shut -down-ar-2208703/ (accessed January 17, 2012).

6. Carole McDonnell, "Manifesting Maggie's Law," *Sleep Review*, http://www.sleeppreviewmag.com/issues/articles/2004-01_06.asp (accessed January 17, 2012).

7. National Sleep Foundation, "1.9 Million Drivers Have Fatigue-Related Car Crashes or Near Misses Each Year," November 2, 2009, http://www.sleepfoundation.org/article/press-release/19-million -drivers-have-fatigue-related-car-crashes-or-near-misses-each-year (accessed October 28, 2011).

8. Benjamin Franklin, *Poor Richard's Almanack* (New York: Skyhorse Publishing, 2007), 13.

CHAPTER 3
KEY 3: FAITH IS A MOVING EXPERIENCE: EXERCISE!

1. Centers for Disease Control, National Diabetes Fact Sheet, 2011, http://www.cdc.gov/diabetes/pubs/pdf/ndfs_2011.pdf (accessed November 1, 2011).

CHAPTER 4
KEY 4: GREAT HEALTH IN THE GREAT OUTDOORS: BREATHE FRESH AIR

1. Centers for Disease Control, "Health Effects of Secondhand Smoke," http://www.cdc.gov/tobacco/data_statistics/fact_sheets/secondhand_ smoke/health_effects/ (accessed November 2, 2011).

2. WebMD, "Effects of Secondhand Smoke," http://www.webmd.com/ smoking-cessation/effects-of-secondhand-smoke (accessed November 2, 2011).

3. US Department of Health and Human Services, "The Health Consequences of Involuntary Exposure to Tobacco Smoke," 2006, http://www.surgeongeneral.gov/library/secondhandsmoke/report/ executivesummary.pdf (accessed November 2, 2011).

CHAPTER 5
KEY 5: GREAT HEALTH IN THE GREAT OUTDOORS: SUNSHINE

1. Mary Brophy Marcus, "Make Your Day Better With Vitamin D," *USA Today*, November 8, 2011, http://yourlife.usatoday.com/health/story/2011-11-08/Make-your-day-better-with-vitamin-D/51113614/1 (accessed January 17, 2012).

2. News Medical, "Researchers Say Health Benefits of Sunshine Outweigh the Skin Cancer Risk and Might Help You Live Longer," http://www.news-medical.net/news/2008/01/07/34041.aspx (accessed November 3, 2011).

3. Johns Hopkins Medicine, "Broccoli Sprout-Derived Extract Protects Against Ultraviolet Radiation," October 22, 2007, http://www.hopkinsmedicine.org/news/media/releases/Broccoli_SproutDerived_Extract_Protects_Against_Ultraviolet_Radiation (accessed January 17, 2012).

4. American Cancer Society, "Skin Cancer Facts," http://www.cancer.org/Cancer/CancerCauses/SunandUVExposure/skin-cancer-facts (accessed November 3, 2011).

5. Johns Hopkins Medicine, "Broccoli Sprout-Derived Extract Protects Against Ultraviolet Radiation."

CHAPTER 6
KEY 6: BRING FORTH FRUIT

1. C. Bernard Gesch et al., "Influence of Supplementary Vitamins, Minerals and Essential Fatty Acids on the Antisocial Behaviour of Young Adult Prisoners," *British Journal of Psychiatry* 181 (2002): 22–28, http://www.ifbb.org.uk/files/Gesch_et_al_2002_British_Journal_of_Psychiatry.pdf (accessed February 21, 2012).

CHAPTER 11
YOUR HEALTH IS YOUR CHOICE. CHOOSE LIFE!

1. Goodreads.com, "Hippocrates Quotes," http://www.goodreads.com/author/quotes/248774.Hippocrates (accessed January 18, 2012).

2. Rex Beach, "Modern Miracle Men," US Senate Document No. 264, http://www.senate.gov/reference/resources/pdf/modernmiraclemen.pdf (accessed February 21, 2012).

CHAPTER 12
DR. DON'S EASY REFERENCE GUIDE FOR COMMON HEALTH PROBLEMS

1. MedPage Today, "FDA Advisers Recommend Black Box Warning for ADHD Drugs" by Peggy Peck, February 9, 2006, http://www.medpagetoday.com/ProductAlert/Prescriptions/2650 (accessed January 18, 2012).

2. Alzheimer's Association, "2011 Alzheimer's Disease Fact and Figures," http://www.alz.org/documents_custom/2011_Facts_Figures_Fact_Sheet.pdf (accessed January 18, 2012).

3. Ibid.

4. Ibid.

5. Carl Elliott, "Create a Disease to Market a New Drug," Kevinmd.com, http://www.kevinmd.com/blog/2011/01/create-disease-market-drug.html (accessed January 19, 2012).

6. G. Roberts, N. Patel, F. Levi-Schaffer, P. Habibi, and G. Lack, "Food Allergy as a Risk Factor for Life-Threatening Asthma in Childhood: A Case-Controlled Study," *Journal of Allergy and Clinical Immunology* 112 (2003).

7. Garth L. Nicolson, "Chronic Fatigue Illness," http://www.immed.org/illness/fatigue_illness_research.html (accessed February 29, 2012).

8. Michael Guthrie, "Mycoplasmas—the Missing Link in Fatiguing Illnesses," *Alternative Medicine*, September 2000, as viewed at ProHealth.com, http://www.prohealth.com/library/showarticle.cfm?libid=7933 (accessed January 18, 2012).

9. Ibid.

10. National Institute of Neurologic Disorders and Stroke, "Questions and Answers About Stroke" http://www.ninds.nih.gov/disorders/stroke/stroke_backgrounder.htm(accessed January 18, 2012).

11. Rock Institute, "Cholesterol: Too High or Too Low?", http://www.therockinstitute.com/rock/wellness-center/articles/article4.pdf (accessed Februray 29, 2012).

12. The Women's Surgery Center, "Endometriosis," http://www.thewomenssurgerycenter.com/endometriosis.htmr (accessed February 21, 2012).

13. Obesity.org, http://www.obesity.org/education/office-management
-of-obesity.htm (accessed January 19, 2012).

14. Centers for Disease Control and Prevention, "Heart Disease Is
the Number One Cause of Death," http://www.cdc.gov/features/
heartmonth/ (accessed January 19, 2012).

15. American Heart Association, "About Diabetes," http://www.heart
.org/HEARTORG/Conditions/Diabetes/AboutDiabetes/About
-Diabetes_UCM_002032_Article.jsp#.T0QMTXkVltg (accessed
February 21, 2012).

16. Ministry Health Care, "Diabetes and Heart Disease," http://
ministryhealth.org/documents/Corporate/HC_Diabetes.pdf
(accessed March 5, 2012).

ABOUT THE AUTHOR

Don VerHulst, MD, received his BS in zoology at the University of Michigan in 1978 and his MD from Wayne State University School of Medicine in 1982. After graduating from medical school, he realized that his continual fast-food diet and late-night study habits had taken a serious physical toll on his body. As he struggled with his stressful, demanding career, the adage "physician, heal thyself" took on a whole new meaning. When he accepted Christ into his heart, though, he felt that every page of the Bible was speaking to him about God's promises of health and wellness for every believer. This launched an intense study of the divine health principles in God's Word from a physician's viewpoint. What he found amazed him. These simple, practical insights inspired Dr. Don's *Do This and Live Healthy.*

Today Dr. Don embraces the naturopathic philosophy of health and has dedicated his life to teaching the principles of preventive medicine. His mission is to share God's simple, effective biblical health plan with as many people as possible. He lectures in schools, churches, and other organizations, and on television and radio programs across the country.

Dr. Don also loves spending time at home with his wife, Susan, who has hosted a Christian radio program for the last twenty years. She is an avid supporter of her husband's work in the health and nutrition field. Together they spend lots of quality time with their four children, Donnie, Aidon, Jaclyn, and Vivian. Dr. Don also enjoys cooking natural foods and working on his music.

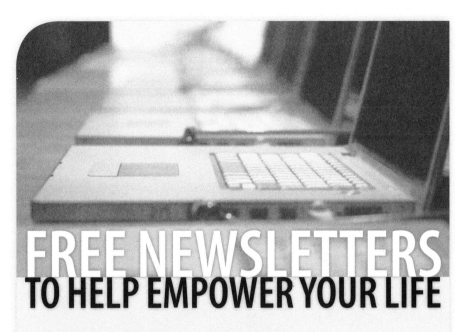

FREE NEWSLETTERS
TO HELP EMPOWER YOUR LIFE

Why subscribe today?

❏ **DELIVERED DIRECTLY TO YOU.** All you have to do is open your inbox and read.

❏ **EXCLUSIVE CONTENT.** We cover the news overlooked by the mainstream press.

❏ **STAY CURRENT.** Find the latest court rulings, revivals, and cultural trends.

❏ **UPDATE OTHERS.** Easy to forward to friends and family with the click of your mouse.

CHOOSE THE E-NEWSLETTER THAT INTERESTS YOU MOST:

- Christian news
- Daily devotionals
- Spiritual empowerment
- And much, much more

SIGN UP AT: **http://freenewsletters.charismamag.com**

8178